Access Your Online Support Material

Harmful Substances is accompanied by a number of printable online materials, designed to ensure this resource best supports your professional needs.

Go to https://resourcecentre.routledge.com/speechmark and click on the cover of this book.

Answer the question prompt using your copy of the book to gain access to the online content.

Harmful Substances

This book goes beyond the surface-level 'just say no' approach, offering deep insights into the real reasons young people may turn to harmful substances and exploring the complex factors – such as coping with trauma, mental health struggles or feelings of inadequacy – that influence these decisions.

Timely and relevant for all educators teaching Personal, Social, Health, Economics (PSHE) education in secondary school, the book provides practical teaching tips, safeguarding guidance and strategies for creating a supportive and inclusive classroom, as well as informative and engaging lesson plans that empower students to make healthier and more informed choices. Supporting a spiral curriculum, it integrates subjects including mental health, science, English and maths, offering a holistic, interdisciplinary approach to learning about harmful substances. This book is not just about prevention teaching – it's about creating a lasting, positive impact on young lives that they can carry on into adulthood.

Created to support all teachers, particularly those new to the subject or who are non-specialists, *Harmful Substances* provides crucial information and knowledge that will ensure effective and impactful classroom sessions.

Nicole Campbell is an educator and PSHE specialist with experience as Senior Subject Lead and Mental Health Lead. She develops Creative Power Education to support young people in exploring identity, resilience, and wellbeing in schools and communities.

PSHE Toolkit

Series Coordinator: Sophie-Lauren McPhee

The PSHE Toolkit Series is a comprehensive companion for delivering engaging and effective Personal, Social, Health and Economic education in secondary schools.

Supporting Your PSHE Teaching Journey

Teaching PSHE effectively requires both expertise and practical resources that work in real classrooms. We understand the challenges you face: limited planning time, diverse student needs, and the pressure to deliver meaningful lessons that make a genuine impact on young people's lives. That's why we've created this series.

Each toolkit provides everything you need to confidently teach key PSHE topics, from Relationships and Sex Education to Financial Literacy and Careers. Whether you're a PSHE specialist or a form tutor covering occasional lessons, these resources will save you time while enhancing your teaching.

What Makes These Toolkits Special?

Each book in the series follows a consistent, user-friendly format that includes:

- Clear explanations of the topic's importance and links to statutory guidance
- Practical teaching tips, including handling sensitive questions and ensuring inclusivity
- Ready-to-use lesson plans for each Key Stage with engaging, varied activities
- Tutor time activities that reinforce learning in shorter sessions
- Assessment tools to track and evidence student progress
- Carefully selected signposting to quality resources and further reading

The activities incorporate proven teaching strategies which encourage students to develop their listening and communication skills, consolidate their knowledge and ask questions, designed to deepen understanding and develop crucial life skills.

Supporting Every Student

These toolkits draw on evidence to encourage a safe, inclusive learning environment where all students can explore important topics, develop critical thinking skills, and prepare for the challenges and opportunities of adolescent and adult life.

Whether you're addressing Relationships, Mental Well-being, Personal Safety, or any of our other carefully selected topics, you'll find practical, thoughtful resources that respect your expertise while saving you valuable time.

Titles available include:

Harmful Substances
Practical Support for Effective Teaching and Learning with Pupils Aged 11–18
Nicole Campbell
2026/Pb: 9781041002703

Harmful Substances

Practical Support for Effective Teaching and Learning with Pupils Aged 11–18

Nicole Campbell

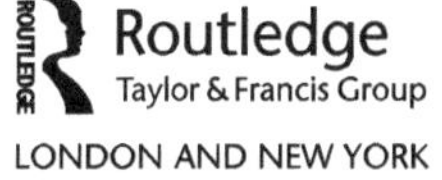

LONDON AND NEW YORK

First published 2026
by Routledge
4 Park Square, Milton Park, Abingdon, Oxon OX14 4RN

and by Routledge
605 Third Avenue, New York, NY 10158

Routledge is an imprint of the Taylor & Francis Group, an informa business

For Product Safety Concerns and Information please contact our EU representative GPSR@taylorandfrancis.com. Taylor & Francis Verlag GmbH, Kaufingerstraße 24, 80331 München, Germany.

British Library Cataloguing-in-Publication Data
A catalogue record for this book is available from the British Library

ISBN: 978-1-041-00286-4 (hbk)
ISBN: 978-1-041-00270-3 (pbk)
ISBN: 978-1-003-60899-8 (ebk)

DOI: 10.4324/9781003608998

Typeset in Optima
by Apex CoVantage, LLC

Access the Support Material: https://resourcecentre.routledge.com/speechmark

Contents

Preface

Teaching PSHE isn't just about delivering information. It's about holding space for young people to explore who they are, what they value and how they relate to the world around them. This work requires care, reflection and responsibility. As you begin this book, I want to welcome you in with both challenge and reassurance because both are essential for meaningful practice.

This book focuses on harmful substances, a topic that can raise strong opinions, uncomfortable truths and personal stories in both pupils and staff. This is why it matters so much. If we want to help our pupils make informed, safe and empowered decisions, we have to be willing to engage with these complexities, not shy away from them.

One of the most important factors in any PSHE lesson is the **relationship between the teacher and their pupils**. This relationship sets the tone. In this subject, especially when dealing with issues like alcohol, vaping, smoking or drug use, it's vital that pupils feel seen, supported and safe. But 'safe' doesn't mean familiar or informal. Pupils should never see us as their friends or feel free to cross boundaries in how they speak to or around us. Instead, our message should be clear: *I care about you, and my job is to keep you safe.*

When I introduce this motto in the classroom, I always remind pupils that anyone under 18 is considered a child which means that we, as the adults, have a safeguarding duty. When the pupils hear that, it often brings smiles to faces. I even see reaffirming nods from some pupils. It gives them a sense of containment. Deep down, most pupils want to feel protected in all areas of their life, even if they don't say it out loud. But alongside that, they also want to be **trusted, heard and respected**, and it's our responsibility to balance those two things.

Consistency of staff, clear boundaries and compassionate professionalism all help build the trust that PSHE relies on.

We also have to remember that **we're not teaching in isolation**. The responsibility for PSHE lies with the whole school community. It should be part of a shared language, a consistent culture. Ideally, it includes open communication with parents and carers, as well as an understanding of the wider community context. Substance use doesn't begin and end in the classroom. It is shaped by family, media, peers and society. If we work collaboratively, we offer pupils synchronised messages and a stronger support system.

At the heart of this work is **self-awareness**. If we're going to help our pupils challenge stigma, shame and social pressures, we have to be doing the same work ourselves. I've seen unconscious bias show up in so many settings: assumptions about which pupils might be using substances or judgemental tones creeping into discussions without us realising. We must hold ourselves accountable for that. The harm that comes from stereotyping or singling out young people is real, and it's also preventable.

As teachers, we need to be actively **reflecting on our own thoughts, beliefs and biases**. That means asking: *Why do I think this? What am I assuming? Whose experience am I focusing on here?* It also means continuing to **educate ourselves**, especially about addiction, trauma and social inequality. Learning about different perspectives and histories helps us understand the full picture and helps us respond to our pupils with empathy, not judgement.

We also need to look inward. There are many forms of addiction in society today. Some visible, some less so. When we begin to reflect honestly on our own relationship with substances, habits or even emotional coping strategies, we become better at understanding others. Empathy begins with humility. You don't need to be perfect. You just need to be willing to notice, unlearn and grow.

This brings us to the importance of **adaptation**. The lesson plans in this book have been designed to be clear, engaging and flexible. They don't contain specific adaptations for special educational needs and disabilities (SEND), English as an additional language (EAL) or any other specific learner group. That's intentional because **you know your pupils best**. As the practitioner, it's your responsibility to adapt content, language and delivery to meet the needs of the pupils in front of you. This includes pupils with

SEND, pupils with learning differences and those who may need emotional or cognitive scaffolding.

In practice, this means:

- Breaking learning down into manageable chunks.
- Pre-teaching vocabulary.
- Offering visual aids or alternative formats.
- Checking for understanding.
- Giving multiple ways to engage: discussion, quiet reflection, drawing or short writing.

You're not expected to do this perfectly. But you are expected to do it thoughtfully. Inclusion isn't a box to tick, it's a mindset. The earlier you build it into your planning, the more natural it becomes.

Another key part of inclusive practice is being **trauma-aware**. For many young people, substance use isn't just a topic, it is part of their lived experience. They may have a parent or sibling who struggles with addiction. They may have lost someone to substance misuse. They may be navigating trauma quietly, without anyone knowing.

So we must tread gently. Avoid using graphic imagery or scare tactics. They don't work, and they can retraumatise our pupils (PSHE Association, 2016). Avoid using shaming language, moralising or a tone that blames. Don't let discussions become unregulated or personal in ways that feel unsafe. Instead, keep the environment structured, respectful and calm. Give pupils the right to step away and check in after sessions. Make it clear that they are never expected to share their personal experiences.

And don't forget to **safeguard yourself**, too. If you've experienced trauma or loss connected to substances or if you have your own history with addiction, give yourself the care and space you need. Talk to your safeguarding lead if you're unsure. You can't support others well if you're overwhelmed or triggered yourself.

Why Did I Write This Book?

I wanted a challenge. My motivation to write this book was to become even better at a topic I knew well, but I also considered how I could help someone teach it with all of its sensitivities. I noticed that teachers feel they have to be experts to teach substance education. They worry about lacking subject knowledge, including definitions and legal consequences. Some may even have personal struggles with drugs or alcohol, which can make engaging with the material and pupils more difficult. This book offers guidance and confidence boosters.

From my experience, honesty and humour, combined with respect and good listening, work really well in classrooms. These qualities help create trust and connection with pupils. I hope this book helps teachers relax and use these qualities to simply talk with their pupils. Even if they don't finish a lesson plan, as long as a good discussion happens, that's a successful outcome. This topic matters deeply to me because of the many young people today who lack support and guidance. I hope this work inspires and builds confidence in teachers and provides the education that pupils truly need.

This book aligns closely with the UK's RSHE (Relationships, Sex and Health Education) guidance, supporting the statutory framework that encourages schools to provide accurate, age-appropriate education about substances. It also reflects international safeguarding principles by promoting a safe, respectful and inclusive learning environment where young people's well-being and protection are central. Throughout, the focus remains on empowering teachers to deliver substance education confidently and sensitively, ensuring pupils receive the knowledge and support they need to make informed decisions.

Finally, a word about **statutory guidance**. Yes, it matters. And yes, we must meet it, but we should not treat it as a ceiling. The guidance sets out the minimum, and we can, and should, go further. That means tailoring content to your cohort, making lessons meaningful for your context and going beyond compliance into **real, impactful education**.

In this book, you'll find lesson plans that are structured, flexible and grounded in both evidence and real classroom practice. But your relationship with your pupils and your professional reflection, that's where the real learning happens.

Let's approach this work with the seriousness it deserves and the compassion it demands.

You've got this!

1 Introduction

Substance education is an essential part of the PSHE curriculum. It is not simply about informing pupils about different substances but also about equipping them with the knowledge and tools to make informed decisions throughout their lives. Even if they are not currently exposed to drugs or alcohol, the skills they develop through this education will be invaluable in the future. Whether they encounter substances themselves or need to support a friend or family member, a strong foundation in substance education ensures they are prepared to navigate these challenges safely and responsibly.

Introducing substance education from a young age is crucial. By laying the foundations early, we help pupils build resilience and develop the confidence to make informed choices. The aim is to instil lifelong skills, not just to keep them safe while they are young, but also to ensure they have the knowledge and strategies to protect themselves well into adulthood. The reality is that without structured education in school, many pupils will not receive this information elsewhere.

Teaching Realistic Strategies

The pressures young people face today are immense. Social influence, peer pressure and media portrayals all contribute to how they perceive substance use. It is not enough to simply teach them to 'say no,' we must provide them with the skills to actively resist harmful influences and navigate high-pressure situations.

Substance education should focus on more than just identifying different substances and discussing their dangers. While knowledge

DOI: 10.4324/9781003608998-1

is important, pupils also need the tools to build resilience, develop critical thinking skills and strengthen their ability to make choices that align with their well-being. Encouraging pupils to reflect on their personal values and long-term goals helps them recognise the consequences of their decisions. When they understand the real-life impact of substance use, not just in terms of health but also in terms of relationships, academic performance and future opportunities, they are better equipped to make informed decisions.

One of the key reasons substance education is so important is because of the many misconceptions that pupils hold. Young people are constantly exposed to information, whether from peers, social media or even family members, and not all of it is accurate. Without proper guidance, they may believe myths such as 'vaping is completely harmless' or 'weed isn't addictive.' These misconceptions can lead to risky behaviour and poor decision-making.

It is essential that we acknowledge where pupils may be getting their information from and actively challenge any misinformation. Encouraging open discussions in the classroom allows pupils to voice their thoughts and question what they may have heard elsewhere. By fostering critical thinking, we empower pupils to assess information for themselves rather than blindly accepting what they are told by others.

Understanding the Adolescent Brain and Risk-Taking Behaviour

During adolescence, the brain goes through major changes, especially in the frontal lobe, the part that helps with planning, self-control, managing emotions and processing new information. This area is slowly maturing, becoming more efficient and specialised over time, a process known as 'neuromaturation' (Squeglia et al., 2009). But substance use can interrupt this development. Studies show that teenagers who drink heavily tend to have smaller prefrontal cortex volumes than those who don't, with the effect being stronger in girls. The impact is even greater for those using both alcohol and marijuana. These changes can make it harder for young people to control their emotions, weigh risks and make good decisions. These are skills that are still maturing and often struggle to keep up with the stronger pull of emotions and rewards.

However other researchers suggest that adolescent brain development, which generally happens between the ages of 10 and 24, is shaped by a mix of factors. Genetics definitely play a part, but so do the environment and any challenges faced before or after birth. Things like nutrition, sleep habits and even medical treatments during early childhood – think medications or surgeries – can all impact how the brain grows. On top of that, stress, whether physical, mental, financial or emotional, can affect development too. It's really important to remember that substance use, like caffeine, nicotine and alcohol, as well as hormonal changes from puberty, all influence how the adolescent brain matures (Arain et al., 2013).

As teachers, knowing how the brain develops helps us teach about substances with more empathy and real impact. Instead of just telling young people to 'just say no,' we can show them how substances affect their growing brains and how these chemicals affect their ability to think clearly, handle stress and judge risks. This isn't just about facts; it's about helping pupils make sense of their feelings and impulses. When they understand why they might be drawn to risky choices, they're better equipped to pause, reflect and make safer decisions.

In class, we can bring this to life with relatable examples, hands-on brain models or conversations about the difference between emotional reactions and logical thinking. Giving pupils this insight changes the conversation from blame or fear to one of awareness, emotional intelligence, responsibility and thoughtful decision-making.

The Changing Landscape of Substance Use

In today's society, substance use is evolving. The landscape of substance use among young people is changing all the time, and it can be hard for teachers to keep up, especially when trends are influenced by social media, peer culture or easy access to misleading information online. That's why it's so important that we, as teachers, stay informed and up to date. Two excellent places to start are the **DSM Foundation**, who offer free, evidence-based resources and CPD for schools, and **Talk to Frank**, which is a clear, non-judgemental source of information on drugs and their effects. They can help you feel more confident and better prepared to answer pupils' questions with clarity and care.

Many young people experiment with substances in social settings, often alongside adults who normalise the behaviour. In some environments, using certain substances is seen as 'just part of having fun' rather than something dangerous or morally questionable. The problem is that the risks often do not become apparent until something goes wrong. It is our role as teachers to ensure that pupils do not have to learn these lessons the hard way. Substance education should never be an afterthought in schools. It is a vital part of safeguarding young people, helping them to develop the confidence and skills to navigate a world where substance use is a reality. By providing them with accurate information, challenging misconceptions and giving pupils practical strategies to resist negative influences, we empower them to make informed, responsible choices.

Our goal is not just to prevent substance use but also to prepare pupils for the pressures they may face now and in the future. When we teach substance education effectively, we are not just protecting young people in the short term, we are also giving them the tools to lead safer, healthier and more informed lives.

Addressing the Needs of All Pupils: Knowledge, Decision-Making and Life Skills

This book aims to help you address the needs of all pupils, recognising that every pupil is different. When teaching substance education, it is crucial to consider these differences and ensure that all pupils, regardless of background or ability, can engage with the topic in a meaningful way. Before delivering any substance education lesson, there are three key areas to consider: knowledge, decision-making and life skills. Each of these plays a vital role in how pupils absorb, process and apply what they learn.

Knowledge

Not all pupils will come to a lesson with the same level of understanding. Some will know very little, while others may have an in-depth awareness of different substances, either through personal experience, exposure within their communities or through social media. I once taught a pupil who could name over 20 different strains of 'skunk' weed. While there was no evidence that they had personally used them, their extensive knowledge was a safeguarding concern. This highlights why it is essential to assess pupils' prior knowledge at the start of a lesson. Simple strategies like asking open-ended questions, observing their written responses or circulating the room to listen to discussions can provide valuable insights into their understanding. It is also crucial to support pupils with special educational needs and disabilities. Some may struggle with abstract concepts, making it important to use pictorial resources alongside terminology to aid comprehension. Providing clear, structured explanations with visual aids can help ensure that all pupils feel included and are able to engage fully with the material.

Decision-Making

Effective decision-making is a critical skill in substance education, but some pupils may find it harder than others to make informed choices. This is particularly relevant for those with learning difficulties or conditions that impact their cognitive processing, impulse control or ability to assess risks. Some pupils may even have undiagnosed needs that affect their decision-making abilities. To support all pupils, lessons should include structured decision-making exercises, such as role-playing scenarios or guided discussions. In some cases, targeted 1:1 or small-group interventions may be beneficial, particularly for pupils who need additional support in developing these skills. By explicitly teaching decision-making as a skill, we can empower pupils to think critically and make choices that align with their well-being.

Life Skills

Every pupil can benefit from learning life skills, but for some, these lessons are particularly crucial. Young carers, for example, may already have responsibilities beyond their years, while other pupils may have experienced circumstances that forced them to grow up quickly. It is essential to work closely with the pastoral team to identify any pupils who may require additional care and sensitivity when discussing substance-related topics. At the same time, we must never assume that all pupils have limited experience with these issues. Some may have witnessed substance use in their families or communities, and it is vital that they do not feel judged or shamed during lessons. Creating a safe, non-judgemental space where pupils feel comfortable discussing these topics is key to ensuring they engage with the material in a way that is meaningful and supportive. By considering knowledge, decision-making and life skills, we can ensure that substance education is accessible, relevant and effective for all pupils, regardless of their individual circumstances.

Reflection Point

Before teaching substance education, it's important to reflect on our own beliefs and assumptions about young people and substance use. Misconceptions can shape the way we approach this topic and impact how effectively we engage pupils. Here are some questions for you to consider:

- What misconceptions might I have about substance use among young people?
- Do I assume that only certain types of pupils are at risk of substance misuse?
- How might media portrayals or my own experiences influence my views on this issue?
- How can I ensure that my teaching remains factual, balanced and free from personal bias?

Take a moment to consider how these reflections might impact your teaching. What steps can you take to ensure your approach is open, non-judgemental and evidence-based?

Understanding 'Harmful Substances'

Before we can effectively teach the topic of harmful substances, we must fully understand what the term means in the context of health, safety and substance education. It is a broad and complex concept, and it is essential that we define it in a way that is appropriate for young people, ensuring that they can engage with the material in a meaningful and age-appropriate way.

The European Commission defines a hazardous substance as 'any material that can cause harm to you directly or indirectly' and 'anything which has the potential to cause injury or damage to people.' This broad definition reminds us that harmful substances are not limited to illegal drugs but include a wide range of everyday substances that can pose risks to health. Understanding this distinction is crucial when educating pupils, as many may assume that only illegal substances are harmful. One of the key aims of substance education is to help pupils categorise harmful substances effectively. This allows them to understand that harm can come from both legal and illegal substances and that some dangers are less obvious than others.

Harmful substances are everywhere. They exist in our food, drinks, air and even the products we use daily. For example, pollutants such as microplastics have been found in the human body, raising concerns about their long-term effects. This challenges the common assumption that harmful substances only come in the form of drugs, alcohol or cigarettes. By helping pupils broaden their perspective, we encourage critical thinking and informed decision-making about what they consume and are exposed to in their environment.

Pupils today tend to think deeply and question societal norms. They may ask, 'If cigarettes and alcohol are harmful, why are they legal?' These types of discussions provide excellent opportunities for debate and deeper understanding. Encouraging pupils to explore why certain substances are regulated rather than banned helps them engage with important topics such as public health policy, government decision-making and corporate influence. Helping pupils understand what makes a substance harmful is key to empowering them to make safer choices. A simple definition, 'any substance that you ingest into your body that can cause harm,' is a useful starting point, but it can also lead to insightful discussions. For example, pupils may raise issues of allergies or the risks of passive smoking, which are less obvious but still significant health concerns.

It is also essential to challenge assumptions about appearance and safety. Many substances do not look harmful, yet they can be incredibly dangerous. For example, weed gummies often resemble ordinary sweets, making them particularly risky for young people who may consume them without realising the potential effects. Discussing these hidden dangers helps pupils become more aware of how substances are marketed and consumed.

Another critical aspect of this discussion is the misconception that natural means safe. Many pupils assume that because something is natural, organic or plant-based, it must be good for them. However, this is not always the case. For example, some poisonous berries may look like edible fruit but can be lethal if consumed. Similarly, certain mushrooms found in the wild are toxic and can cause severe illness or death. Teaching pupils to be cautious about what they ingest, whether in nature, at home or in social settings, is an important life skill that could potentially save lives.

By helping pupils develop a broad perspective on harmful substances, we equip them with the knowledge to question, analyse and make informed decisions. The goal is not to instil fear but to encourage awareness and responsibility. Understanding that harm does not only come from illegal drugs but also from everyday substances, environmental factors and even natural sources allows pupils to navigate their world with greater confidence and caution. Encouraging open discussions, debate and critical thinking will help pupils see the complexities of substance use and regulation. By fostering this deeper understanding, we empower young people to take control of their own health and well-being in a world where harmful substances, both visible and hidden, are an unavoidable reality.

The Emergence of New Substances and Trends

Statistics can be incredibly useful in understanding trends in substance use, but it is also important to consider their limitations. Cases of substance use may go unreported, meaning that the official figures may not tell the full story. As teachers, we should encourage pupils to think critically about data, questioning where statistics come from, what they represent and what might be missing.

The following statistics are based on findings from the UK Government's Office for Health Improvement and Disparities report (January 2024). If you are teaching outside the United Kingdom, it is worth researching local or regional data to ensure the information is relevant to your pupils. According to the report, cannabis remains the most common substance (87%) that young people seek treatment for. This is a significant statistic, highlighting the need for cannabis education to be a key focus in substance education. While other substances are also prevalent, cannabis stands out as the most commonly used drug among young people, reinforcing the importance of educating pupils about its risks, effects and potential long-term consequences.

The report also states that

- 44% of young people in treatment reported alcohol-related issues.
- 7% reported problems with ecstasy.
- 9% reported problems with powder cocaine.

This data suggests that alcohol and cannabis use often go hand in hand, meaning that substance education should not treat them in isolation.

There have been changes in the prevalence of certain drugs among young people. The report highlights a decline in the number of young people seeking help for codeine use, which fell from 1.2% in 2020–21 to 0.8% in 2022–23. While this is encouraging, any percentage above zero is still a concern, particularly given the highly addictive nature of codeine. Again, it is worth noting that not all users seek treatment, so the actual number may be higher than reported. However, it is worth considering whether the COVID-19 pandemic contributed to the previous increase in use. A comparative analysis of pre-pandemic and post-pandemic data could help us understand whether these substances were being used as coping mechanisms during periods of lockdown and social isolation.

Other substances, however, are becoming more widely used. The report found that

- The number of young people in treatment for solvent misuse rose significantly, from 329 cases (2.9%) in 2021–22 to 629 cases (5.1%) in 2022–23.

- Reports of ketamine-related problems increased from 512 cases (4.5%) in 2021–22 to 719 cases (5.8%) in 2022–23.

While this report provides insight into existing trends, new substances are constantly emerging, which means teachers must stay informed and keep up to date with the most recent research. One of the most concerning drug trends is 'Spice,' a synthetic cannabinoid that is reported to be far stronger and more addictive than cannabis. Unlike traditional cannabis, Spice can have unpredictable and severe effects, making it particularly dangerous. Similarly, nitrous oxide (laughing gas) is becoming increasingly popular among young people. The casual perception of nitrous oxide as 'harmless fun' means that many young people are unaware of the serious risks associated with it, including oxygen deprivation, nerve damage and even fatal overdoses.

Research from Manchester Metropolitan University (2022) also raised an important concern: if young people are told they can overdose on certain substances, this can sometimes increase their curiosity and make them seek out those drugs. This highlights the delicate balance required in substance education; we must inform pupils without unintentionally promoting interest in dangerous substances.

In recent years, ketamine use has become more visible among young people, a concerning trend that's often overlooked. While ketamine is a licensed medical drug, used as an anaesthetic and for pain management, it's also misused recreationally and sometimes referred to as a 'horse tranquiliser' due to its veterinary uses. When taken outside of a medical setting, ketamine can cause serious long-term harm. One of the most damaging effects is on the bladder. Regular misuse can lead to chronic bladder pain, frequent urination and even permanent damage. In severe cases, there's also a risk of kidney complications.

A BBC article shares the story of Ryan, a young man now being diagnosed for possible kidney failure due to ketamine misuse. He talks openly about the impact it's had on his daily life, including passing blood and needing to urinate repeatedly throughout the day. He's also deeply worried about what this means for his future relationships and the possibility of having children.

It's a stark reminder that substance education isn't about scare tactics, it's about facts. Young people need to know the long-term consequences so they can make informed, respectful decisions about their health and future. Understanding emerging drug trends is crucial in ensuring that substance education remains relevant and effective. The statistics show us that young people are using substances earlier than ever, often in combination with other drugs, and that certain substances, such as solvents and ketamine, are on the rise.

More importantly, substance use is often linked to deeper social and emotional issues, which means that education must go beyond just facts and figures. It must also address the root causes of why young people turn to substances in the first place.

As new drugs continue to emerge, teachers must stay informed.

What This Book Is Not

This book is not designed to scare or shame young people into avoiding substances. We know that outdated approaches based on fear or judgement simply don't work, and in some cases they can actually damage trust or push pupils away from asking for help. You won't find any moralising here. Instead, this book offers a practical, fact-based and reflective approach to teaching about substances, grounded in what young people actually need: knowledge, self-awareness, space to ask questions and tools to make informed choices. This resource also avoids assumptions. It does not assume that every young person is using substances or that none of them are. It doesn't frame drug and alcohol use in extremes, and it avoids stereotypes about who uses what and why.

Instead, lessons are designed to create safe, inclusive classrooms where pupils feel respected, not judged. A place where their experiences, questions and worries are taken seriously. A space where the focus is on building skills, not delivering lectures. If you're a teacher feeling nervous about 'getting it right,' this book is here to support you. You don't have to be a subject expert. You just need to be open, curious and willing to facilitate the conversation.

How Young People Encounter Harmful Substances

Peer influence and social media play a significant role in exposing young people to substances. While family and friends are often seen as the most traditional sources of influence, the modern landscape has evolved. Music, for example, frequently promotes drug and alcohol use in a positive light, making these behaviours seem glamorous or even expected. Experimentation with substances has become increasingly normalised, and social media influencers and celebrities contribute to this by openly showcasing drug and alcohol use.

These figures hold immense power, not just because of their visibility and reach, but also because they make substance use seem casual, fun and without consequence. For many young people, the appeal lies in the fact that their role models, people they admire and aspire to be like, are engaging in these behaviours. This creates two significant risks.

Firstly, young people may feel compelled to imitate what they see online, believing that trying drugs or alcohol is simply part of growing up. The desire to fit in, seek excitement or replicate the lifestyles they observe on social media can lead them to experiment with substances. Secondly, excessive social media use itself can contribute to poor mental health, particularly when combined with sleep deprivation and the pressures of 'FOMO' (fear of missing out). In some cases, this decline in mental well-being may increase the likelihood of turning to substances as a coping mechanism.

This book is part of a wider PSHE Toolkit series focused on harmful substances, but substance education cannot exist in isolation. To fully support young people, we need to ensure they understand the broader connections, how substance misuse links to physical health, mental health, peer pressure and online influences. You will notice references throughout this book to other PSHE topics, reinforcing the interconnected nature of these issues. As a PSHE specialist, I have learned that true expertise comes from recognising how all these areas overlap because, ultimately, PSHE is about equipping young people with essential life skills.

Given the impact of social media, it is crucial that we speak with pupils to understand what platforms they use, how often they use them and the content they engage with. Once we have this insight, we can turn the tables, empowering pupils to become positive influencers themselves.

Encouraging them to create social media campaigns that promote healthy choices, resilience and critical thinking can be an incredibly effective way to challenge harmful narratives online.

Ultimately, we must recognise and address the ways young people encounter harmful substances. Open discussions are key, as they allow us to understand their world before stepping in with guidance. More importantly, we must harness the power of positive peer influence, counteracting the risks posed by social media and peer pressure with proactive, empowering strategies. By doing so, we can help pupils become social advocates, using their voices to support and inspire others rather than being passively influenced by harmful trends.

Reflection Point

Take the time now to think about

- How often do I discuss social media influence with my pupils?
- Could I incorporate more conversations about digital literacy and substance exposure in my lessons?

Why This Topic Is Urgent in Schools Today

The fact that **14,352 children and young people** were in alcohol and drug treatment between April 2023 and March 2024 represents a sharp **16% rise from the previous year**. On the surface, this could feel quite alarming and rightly so. For those of us working in education, it suggests that substance-related harms are not abstract possibilities but very real issues affecting a growing number of the children we teach (Office for Health Improvement & Disparities, 2024).

While the number is still **41% lower than the peak in 2008 to 2009**, this recent rise should still serve as a red flag. It's a reminder that young people today are facing complex pressures and that harmful substance use continues to be one of the ways some are coping with what's going on in their lives, whether that's stress, trauma, mental health difficulties or social influences. The increase might also reflect improved access to services and growing awareness of available support, which is a step in the right direction. But it still tells us that more young people are reaching a point where specialist help is needed.

For teachers, this trend highlights the importance of **early, preventative education**, not just to raise awareness, but also to build pupils' confidence, resilience and sense of self-worth before issues escalate. It reinforces why we need a **whole-school approach** to harmful substance education, moving beyond scare tactics and offering honest, inclusive and supportive teaching. It also shows why **ongoing training** for staff is vital, so we're confident in spotting signs of concern and responding with care, not judgement.

Ultimately, we can't assume that substance misuse is something that happens 'elsewhere' or only affects a certain type of pupil. This rise reminds us that it could be happening in our schools and our classrooms, and it's our responsibility to be ready (Office for Health Improvement & Disparities, 2024).

There are several reasons why cannabis remains so prevalent among young people. According to the UK Addiction Treatment Centres (2021), cannabis use is often **easy to conceal**, the effects are **widely perceived to be safe** and **society is increasingly accepting** of its use. On top of that, cannabis tends to be **cheaper** than many other substances, making it more accessible. These factors together create a sense of normalisation that can influence young people's choices, especially if they're already feeling under pressure or looking for ways to cope.

What's more concerning is that cannabis isn't the only substance on the rise. **Around 2 in 5** young people (39%) in treatment reported problems with alcohol. There are also increasing numbers of pupils presenting with issues related to **ecstasy** (9%), **powder cocaine** (8%) and, most notably, **ketamine**, which rose significantly from **512 cases in 2021–22 to 1,201 in 2023–24**. For the first time ever, more young people are reporting problems with ketamine than with cocaine. Similarly, **solvent and inhalant misuse**, including **nitrous oxide**, rose from 2.9% to 6.1% in the same timeframe (Office for Health Improvement & Disparities, 2024).

For those of us working in education, these patterns suggest a real need to **update our teaching materials**, stay aware of **emerging substance trends** and create **lesson content** that pupils recognise as relevant to their world. Pupils need accurate information, not just scare stories, about substances they may already be exposed to through friends, social media or popular culture.

This also speaks to the importance of creating a **non-judgemental classroom culture**. If young people perceive us as moralising or dismissive, they're far less likely to engage with us. But if we can show them that we're informed, open and there to support, not shame, then we have a better chance of making a lasting impact.

A particularly concerning aspect of the most recent data is the level of **vulnerability** among the children and young people entering substance misuse treatment. According to the Office for Health Improvement & Disparities (2024), the **most common issue** reported was **early onset of substance use**, with a striking **80%** of young people stating they began using substances **before the age of 15**. This early exposure has serious implications for brain development, risk-taking behaviour and long-term well-being.

For teachers, this statistic is not just a number, it's also a clear call to action. If young people are beginning to experiment with substances so early, then schools cannot afford to delay drug and alcohol education until the later years of secondary school. Education must be **preventative, not reactive**, and delivered in a way that resonates with pupils before risky behaviours take root.

Another significant concern is **poly-drug use**, reported by **56%** of young people in treatment. This suggests that many pupils are not just experimenting with one substance, but are also mixing several, often without fully understanding the combined risks. From a teaching point of view, this reinforces the importance of **fact-based, non-sensationalist** education that clearly explains how different substances interact and the potential consequences of combining them.

Perhaps most distressing are the vulnerabilities reported disproportionately by girls. **Self-harming behaviours** were disclosed by **52% of girls** compared to just **17% of boys**, and **9% of girls** reported experiences of **sexual exploitation**, compared to **1.2% of boys** (Office for Health Improvement & Disparities, 2024). These figures highlight a complex intersection between trauma, exploitation and substance use.

As teachers, this reminds us that a young person's substance use may be **a coping strategy** rather than simply a rebellious act. We must always approach the topic with empathy, curiosity and an understanding that **behaviour is communication**. It is a language. Trauma-informed, inclusive practice isn't optional here. It is essential if we are to safeguard our pupils and support their long-term well-being.

Figure 1.1 shows that even at **age 12**, there are **nearly 300 children** (151 girls, 145 boys) already in treatment for substance misuse. By **age 13**, the number has doubled. This reinforces what was said before: this education needs to begin earlier than we might think, and certainly **before Year 9**. The most significant spike happens between **13 and 15 years old**. At 15, there are **3,951 children** in treatment (1,489 girls and 2,462 boys). This is a critical age, when pressure from peers intensifies, independence increases

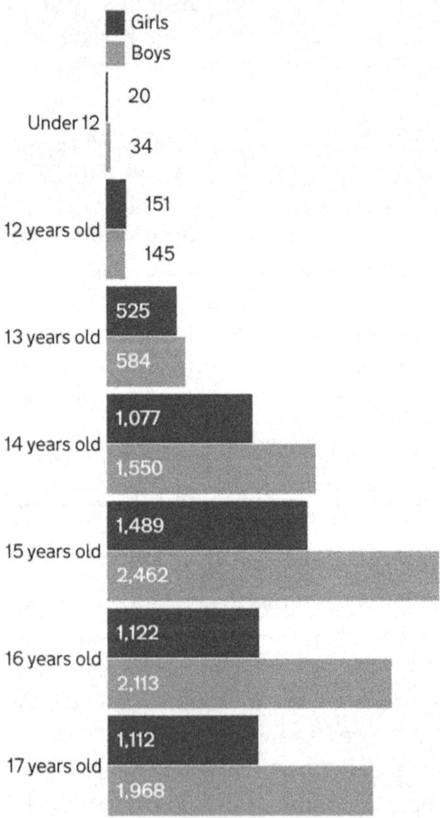

Figure 1.1 Number of children and young people in substance misuse treatment by age and gender (April 2023–March 2024).
Source: Office for Health Improvement & Disparities, 2024

and risk-taking becomes more common. Teachers working with KS4 pupils need to be especially aware that these pupils may be at the **highest risk of harm**, even if they don't outwardly 'present' as such.

While the numbers start fairly even at younger ages, by age 14 and onwards, **boys are much more likely to be in treatment than girls**. For example, at age 15, there are nearly **1,000 more boys than girls** in treatment. This might reflect differences in risk behaviour, access or even how substance use presents. However, we also must consider that **girls may be underrepresented** due to shame or fear of stigma, especially if their substance use is connected to trauma or exploitation, as previously mentioned. However, despite lower treatment numbers, we know from the OHID report (2024) that girls in treatment are more likely to report vulnerabilities like **self-harm** and **sexual exploitation**. This means schools must **actively create safe, trauma-informed spaces** for girls to come forward.

There are some implications from this data that can help us to improve the way we educate about harmful substances in schools:

- **Preventative education should start in upper primary or early secondary**, delivered with sensitivity and clarity, not fear-based messaging. It may also be necessary to have gender-specific approaches. Boys may need targeted work around risk-taking, masculinity and peer pressure. Girls may need emotional safety, assurance of confidentiality and trusted adults they feel safe disclosing to. Non-binary pupils also need the space to feel safe and share openly. All groups benefit from representation, empathy and inclusive discussion.
- These lessons aren't just about knowledge, they're also about **safety**, **identity** and **belonging**. The pupils who are struggling might not say it out loud, but they're more likely to engage when the session feels safe, inclusive and respectful of their reality.

The Link Between Substance Use and Mental Health Issues

Why do people take drugs in the first place? This is an important question to ask because there isn't just one answer. People use substances for different reasons, and some individuals are more vulnerable than others, a topic we will explore later. For now, we will focus on the relationship between substance use and mental health issues.

A common question is: *Does substance use lead to mental health issues, or do mental health issues lead to substance use?* The answer is that both can be true.

Some individuals experience existing mental health issues and turn to drugs or alcohol as a way to self-medicate or cope with how they feel. For example, a young person struggling with anxiety, depression or trauma might use substances in an attempt to numb their emotions or escape their reality. However, while substances might provide temporary relief, they often worsen mental health problems over time, leading to dependency and a cycle of addiction.

Not everyone who starts using substances does so because they are struggling. Some young people begin using substances from a place of happiness and curiosity. For example, someone who is mentally well might experiment with cannabis while spending time with friends. At first, they might laugh, feel relaxed and enjoy the experience. However, prolonged or increased use can lead to paranoia, hopelessness, depression or anxiety. Research suggests that frequent cannabis use is linked to an increased risk of developing psychosis or schizophrenia, particularly in those already vulnerable to mental health conditions (Mental Health Foundation, 2021).

A similar pattern can be seen with alcohol. Drinking might initially be a fun and social experience, helping some young people feel more confident, outgoing or less anxious. However, over time, relying on alcohol to boost self-esteem or suppress emotions can lead to dependency, increased risk-taking behaviour and a decline in mental well-being. Excessive alcohol consumption has been strongly linked to higher rates of depression and anxiety disorders.

It is important for young people to understand that not everyone who starts using substances is already struggling with their mental health. However, they should be aware that prolonged use of harmful substances can lead to serious mental health issues. Additionally, drug addiction itself is classified as a mental health disorder. The *DSM-V* (*Diagnostic and Statistical Manual of Mental Disorders*) recognises substance-related and addictive disorders, reinforcing the fact that addiction is a medical condition, not just a lifestyle choice. By educating young people on these risks, we empower them to make informed choices about their well-being and help them understand the interplay between substance use and mental health.

The Department for Education's guidance on mental health and well-being emphasises that schools must equip pupils with the knowledge and skills to manage their mental health, which includes addressing the risks associated with substance misuse. Teachers should be aware of signs of mental health struggles and substance abuse, and schools must have clear support systems in place to assist pupils.

Reflection Point

Take the time to consider the following:

- What signs of substance use or mental health struggles should I be looking for in my pupils? What support systems are in place at my school for pupils who might be at risk?
- How can I introduce the idea that addiction is a mental health disorder in an age-appropriate and non-judgemental way? What misconceptions might my pupils already have?

The Impact on Education: Attendance, Attainment and Behaviour

Attendance

Substance misuse can have a significant impact on a pupil's attendance. When pupils engage with drugs or alcohol, it can result in them truanting from school for various reasons. They may be absent due to hangovers, recovering from a drug-related illness or simply because they have had a negative experience linked to their substance use. In some cases, pupils may miss school because they are spending time with others who are also engaging in substance misuse.

This poor attendance can create gaps in learning, leaving pupils behind in their education. Missing lessons, assignments and important discussions can quickly lead to them falling behind, which, over time, becomes harder to recover from. Without the support of regular attendance, pupils may struggle to keep up with their peers academically.

Attainment

Substance misuse can also impair cognitive function, making it difficult for pupils to perform at their best. Drugs and alcohol can affect memory, concentration and critical thinking, which in turn can lead to lower academic achievement. For example, pupils may find it harder to study, retain information or engage fully in lessons. In addition, substances can disrupt sleep patterns, which are crucial for cognitive function. Poor sleep can result in tiredness during the school day, affecting the pupil's ability to focus and participate in learning activities. This reduced cognitive capacity leads to lower grades and potentially poor exam performance, undermining the pupil's overall academic potential.

Behaviour

Substance misuse can affect the brain regions that control mood and behaviour, leading to changes in how pupils interact with their peers and teachers. For some, substance use may result in becoming more disruptive, possibly acting out in class or engaging in risky behaviour. For others, the impact may be the opposite, where the pupil becomes more docile or withdrawn. The way substances affect an individual's behaviour can vary widely depending on the person and the substance involved.

The biggest concern, however, is that substance misuse can undermine a pupil's ability to maintain a healthy routine and develop positive relationships with others. It can make it harder for pupils to establish the emotional and social connections they need for success in school and beyond. The impact on relationships, both with peers and teachers, can further isolate the pupil, affecting both their academic and personal growth.

In short, substance misuse can affect a pupil's attendance, academic performance and behaviour, all of which are closely linked to their overall success and well-being in education, and life, in general.

Statutory Guidance and Responsibilities in Schools

As we've just discussed, substance misuse can deeply impact pupils' attendance, academic performance and behaviour. In the United Kingdom, schools have a legal responsibility to address substance misuse as part of their duty to ensure the safety, well-being and education of all pupils. The Department for Education's (DfE) statutory guidance on 'Health and Wellbeing' for schools outlines how substance misuse should be addressed in the curriculum. This includes providing age-appropriate education about the risks of drugs, alcohol and other substances and ensuring pupils are equipped with the knowledge and skills to make informed decisions. Schools are also required to have clear policies for managing substance misuse incidents, ensuring both prevention and support for pupils affected.

It is essential for schools to not only educate pupils about the dangers of substance misuse but also to provide appropriate support services for pupils who are struggling or curious. This may include access to counselling, working with external agencies and providing intervention programmes that address both the mental health and substance misuse of pupils. By adhering to statutory guidance, schools can create a safe, supportive environment that helps mitigate the negative impacts of substance misuse on pupils' educational outcomes.

The Science Behind Harmful Substances

Let's be honest, this part of the topic can feel overwhelming. There is just so much information out there on the health harms of drugs. But as teachers, we don't need to know everything. What we do need is a clear understanding of the key issues so we can support our pupils with confidence and correct misinformation when it arises. According to the Centre for Public Health (2011), the health harms associated with drug use vary depending on the substance and the frequency of use.

You don't have to be a scientist to talk about drugs in PSHE. What helps is having a clear structure and being able to share the facts in a way that makes sense for your pupils. Let's break this down into manageable parts.

Physical Health Effects

One of the most obvious concerns is how drugs affect the body. Some substances can damage vital organs like the heart, lungs, liver and kidneys. Others might increase the risk of long-term conditions or sudden medical emergencies. Some pupils may not realise that drugs can have physical effects that aren't visible straight away. For example, regular cannabis use can affect lung function, and stimulants like MDMA can impact the heart and lead to overheating and dehydration.

There's also the risk of infections if needles are involved, which opens up the conversation about blood-borne viruses like hepatitis and HIV. These are all facts that pupils need to know but may not learn about elsewhere.

Mental Health Effects

This part is especially important because young people often use substances to cope with how they're feeling. But what many don't realise is that certain drugs can actually make those feelings worse in the long run. Cannabis, for example, is often linked with increased anxiety and paranoia. Alcohol can make a low mood feel even heavier the next day. Prolonged use can lead to more serious mental health conditions, including depression or drug-induced psychosis.

It's also worth explaining how some drugs mask emotional pain in the short term but can make mental well-being harder to manage over time.

Cognitive and Behavioural Impact

Substance use can impact brain development, particularly in younger teens. This might affect memory, concentration and the ability to focus in class. It can also affect sleep patterns, which in turn has a knock-on effect on energy levels, attendance and behaviour. Some pupils might appear more withdrawn or more easily agitated without linking it to their substance use.

Dependency and Addiction

This is where things become even more serious. Repeated use of a drug can lead to dependency. That means the person needs more and more of the substance to feel the same effect. Over time, this can lead to addiction, which is recognised as a mental health disorder. It's important to explain to pupils that addiction can happen gradually, and sometimes even with substances they think are low risk, like vaping or codeine.

Substance Overview

Rather than overwhelm pupils with information, it's helpful to focus on the most common substances they might come across:

- Cannabis.
- Alcohol.
- Vapes and e-cigarettes.
- Nitrous oxide (also known as laughing gas).
- Prescription drug misuse (such as codeine).
- Party drugs such as MDMA.

Each of these comes with its own set of risks, so choose which ones are most relevant for your pupils and setting.

When we talk about substance misuse to our pupils, it's not just about warning them about what not to do. It's about helping them understand what's happening to their minds and bodies and giving them tools to make healthy choices. Young people are exposed to a lot of misinformation online, and if we don't step in to educate them properly, they'll turn to unreliable sources.

PSHE is the perfect space for these conversations. It links to mental health, physical health, risk, decision-making and relationships. This isn't a one-off topic. It's a key part of preparing pupils for life.

Reflection Point

Take the time to consider the following:

- How confident do I feel explaining the health harms of substances to my pupils?
- Are there any common myths or misconceptions I need to unlearn or clarify?

Legal and Ethical Considerations

This section of the book is particularly important for non-specialist teachers. Pupils must understand the legal and ethical consequences associated with drug possession, production and supply, and, as teachers, we need to feel confident delivering this content clearly and accurately.

The UK Laws on Drugs, Alcohol and Vaping

According to HM Government, the penalties for drug possession vary depending on the classification of the drug and the circumstances involved, such as the quantity in possession and whether there is any evidence of production or intent to supply.

This area could easily become an entire lesson in itself. And if you're not familiar with how drugs are categorised or the sentencing guidelines, don't worry, you're not alone. Here is a simplified list of drugs currently categorised under Classes A, B and C in the United Kingdom:

Class A

- Cocaine.
- Crack cocaine.
- Ecstasy (MDMA).
- Heroin.

- LSD.
- Magic mushrooms.
- Methadone.
- Methamphetamine (crystal meth).

Class B

- Amphetamines.
- Barbiturates.
- Cannabis.
- Codeine.
- GHB (gamma hydroxybutyrate).
- GBL (gamma-butyrolactone).
- Ketamine.
- Methylphenidate (Ritalin).
- Synthetic cannabinoids.
- Synthetic cathinones (e.g. mephedrone, methoxetamine).

Class C

- Anabolic steroids.
- Benzodiazepines (e.g. diazepam).
- Khat.
- Nitrous oxide (laughing gas).
- Piperazines (e.g. BZP).

There are also temporary class drugs. These are substances that may not yet be formally classified, but which the police are still authorised to seize. These are often fast-tracked to be banned by the government due to emerging risks.

Penalties

- Class A: Possession can result in up to 7 years in prison, an unlimited fine or both. Supplying or producing carries a maximum sentence of life imprisonment, an unlimited fine or both.

- Class B: Possession can result in up to 5 years in prison, an unlimited fine or both. Supplying or producing carries a maximum of 14 years.
- Class C: Possession could lead to up to 2 years in prison, an unlimited fine or both. As with Class B, supplying or producing can lead to up to 14 years in prison.

For pupils under 18, it's also worth noting that the police have the right to inform parents, carers or guardians if they are caught with drugs.

If your pupils ask something you don't know the answer to, it's absolutely fine to say, 'I'm not sure, let's find out together.' This not only models honesty and humility, but also reinforces the idea that learning is lifelong, even for teachers.

Alcohol and Vaping

The law also outlines strict age-related restrictions on alcohol. According to HM Government, it is illegal for

- Anyone to sell alcohol to someone under 18.
- A person under 18 to attempt to buy alcohol.
- An adult to buy or attempt to buy alcohol on behalf of someone under 18.

Young people can also be stopped, fined or even arrested if caught drinking alcohol in public places.

When it comes to vaping, the National Health Service states that it is illegal to sell vape products to anyone under 18 or for adults to purchase them on their behalf. Unfortunately, some vapes sold in the United Kingdom still do not meet safety regulations and may contain dangerously high levels of harmful substances, something young people and teachers should be especially aware of.

When we talk about legal consequences, it is really important to consider how the law impacts young people specifically, as well as the ripple effects this can have on their families. Often, these are the conversations that get missed in school settings. Teachers may not always feel confident discussing legal matters, but it is vital we understand the basics so we can better support our pupils and guide them towards the right help when needed.

Let's start with how the law treats young people differently from adults. In the United Kingdom, if someone under the age of 18 is found in possession of drugs, alcohol or illegal vapes, they may face a different set of consequences compared to adults. These can include being issued a youth caution or a conditional caution. In some cases, they might be referred to a youth offending team. This is usually done to help the young person get support, rather than to punish them. But let's be clear, these records do not just disappear. Even a caution could affect future opportunities, including travel, university applications and employment.

In schools, legal consequences can go hand in hand with disciplinary measures. For example, if a pupil is found with drugs or alcohol on school premises, it could lead to a fixed-term exclusion or even permanent exclusion. In some cases, a pupil might be moved to another school entirely. There are also safeguarding implications. If a young person is suspected of using or being involved with drugs, staff have a duty to act and follow their school's safeguarding procedures.

What about families? The law can touch them too. If a young person is getting into trouble with substances, it can lead to wider investigations into their welfare. This might involve social services stepping in to assess the family situation. In extreme cases, parents or carers could be issued a parenting order, which legally requires them to attend parenting classes or take steps to support their child's behaviour. Aside from legal concerns, there is the emotional impact. Parents might feel guilt, fear or shame, especially if they feel they did not see the signs or do enough to prevent the behaviour. This is why schools need to take a proactive approach. By building strong partnerships with families and making use of local agencies, we can ensure there is a joined-up response. Prevention is always better than reaction.

Ethical Considerations

This part of the chapter is where we really ask: just because something is legal or illegal, does that make it right or wrong? Ethics is all about how we make decisions, especially when those decisions affect others. For young people, understanding the difference between having a *right to choose* and being *responsible for the consequences* is key.

You can explore questions like

- What does it mean to make an *informed* choice?
- How does peer pressure affect someone's ability to choose freely?
- Are young people truly responsible if they don't fully understand the risks involved?
- What about the responsibilities we all have to keep each other safe?

You could bring in real-life classroom discussions here. For example, when discussing vaping or drug use, some pupils might argue that it's 'their body, their choice.' This is where we can gently challenge them, 'yes, you have autonomy, but every choice has a consequence.' If your choice affects your mental health, your schoolwork, your family or your peers, it's no longer just a personal decision. This is also an excellent opportunity to talk about restorative approaches. Instead of punishment alone, how do we help pupils take ownership, learn from mistakes and repair harm? This aligns closely with PSHE's values of empathy, accountability and self-awareness.

Reflection Point

Take the time to consider the following:

- How do I help pupils see the bigger picture of their decisions?
- What classroom strategies can I use to teach empathy, accountability and responsible choice-making?

Addressing Misinformation and Myths

In this section, we are going to explore misinformation around drugs and alcohol misuse. In class discussions, I've often heard pupils speak confidently about what they think they know about certain substances. More often than not, they are sharing things they have heard rather than facts they know for themselves. There's usually a sense of enthusiasm when they talk about it, but the accuracy is not always there. For example, when we discuss cannabis, I sometimes introduce the difference between the natural plant and synthetic forms like skunk. Many pupils do not realise there is a distinction between the two and that these variations can have very different effects on the brain and body.

As teachers, it is important to reflect on how we respond in those moments when a pupil shares something that may not be factually correct. With the rest of the class listening, it is vital we do not unintentionally reinforce misinformation. Rather than shutting down the conversation or correcting them in a way that may feel dismissive, we can use these opportunities to model curiosity and fact-checking.

A really effective approach can be to say something like, 'That's an interesting point, let's look into that together.' This helps pupils see that not knowing everything is fine and that learning is a shared process. It also teaches them how to seek out reliable information, which is a crucial life skill.

Let's encourage pupils to question where their information comes from and to be more critical of the things they hear, especially online or in social settings. Our role is not only to correct misconceptions, but also to help pupils build the confidence and tools they need to do that for themselves.

Reflection Point

Take the time to consider the following:

- How do I usually respond when a pupil shares something that might not be factually correct?
- Do I encourage exploration or shut it down?

In PSHE, one of our key responsibilities is to promote evidence-based knowledge and develop pupils' critical thinking. But here's the challenge: when we introduce common myths around drugs, alcohol or vaping, we risk unintentionally reinforcing them, especially if we're not careful in how we present and explore them.

So how do we tackle myths in a way that strengthens understanding rather than undermining it?

We begin by framing myths not as 'fun facts' or 'shocking truths' but as real examples of misinformation that exist in our communities and online. We can then use these examples to help pupils practise evaluating sources, questioning assumptions and exploring how beliefs are shaped. For instance, when addressing the myth that 'vaping is just flavoured water,' we don't just tell pupils it's incorrect. Instead, we ask them to examine where that message might have come from. Was it advertising? Peer conversation? TikTok? Then, we guide them to find and assess reliable sources, like the NHS or government health advice, and compare what's being said.

This approach helps pupils build the habit of fact-checking, and it teaches them to sit with uncertainty, to ask, 'Do I know this because it's true, or just because I've heard it often?'

Reflection Point

Take the time to consider the following:

- How can I use myths as a gateway to develop pupils' research and reasoning skills, rather than just dismissing them as 'wrong'?

By exploring myths thoughtfully, we're not just correcting misinformation, we're building the tools pupils need to think critically, make informed decisions and become more reflective learners in and beyond the classroom.

Navigating Personal Beliefs and Cultural Sensitivities

While exploring myths and misinformation in PSHE can be a powerful learning opportunity, we also need to be mindful of how these conversations may intersect with pupils' personal beliefs, cultural backgrounds or religious views. Sometimes what we label as a 'myth' may conflict with values that pupils have grown up with or what they've been told by family or community members. This can create discomfort or even tension in the classroom. As teachers, we're not here to dismiss or invalidate pupils' beliefs but rather to provide a safe and respectful space where pupils can examine different perspectives and learn how to engage in critical thinking. This is part of helping them become thoughtful, informed citizens.

When a myth touches on sensitive ground, it's helpful to acknowledge this openly and invite pupils into the process of respectful discussion. You might say something like,

> Some of us may have heard different things about this topic depending on our families or backgrounds, and that's fine. In this lesson, we're going to look at what the evidence says, and we'll explore why different people might believe different things.

This approach not only validates pupils' lived experiences but also helps them practise respectful disagreement and develop empathy. It teaches them that it's possible to question ideas without questioning someone's identity or background.

Reflection Point

Take the time to consider the following:

- How do I currently create space for pupils to bring their own perspectives into lessons, especially when those views may differ from the curriculum or evidence?

By keeping curiosity, kindness and evidence at the heart of these discussions, we can turn potentially uncomfortable moments into meaningful learning experiences and help pupils feel seen, valued and heard.

Working With External Partners

Many schools choose to bring in external organisations to deliver parts of their PSHE curriculum, especially around complex topics like drugs, alcohol or relationships. While these providers can offer specialised knowledge and a fresh voice for pupils, it's important to approach this with care.

Not all external speakers will have a deep understanding of what high-quality, safe and inclusive PSHE looks like. Some may come with lived experience or professional expertise, but that doesn't automatically mean they are equipped to handle sensitive discussions in a way that's developmentally appropriate or aligned with the values of your school.

As teachers, we know that how something is taught is just as important as what is taught.

Before inviting anyone into the classroom, consider asking the following questions:

- Do they understand the principles of safe PSHE delivery, including how to avoid sensationalism or scare tactics?
- Do they respect pupil voice and ensure there is space for questions, reflection and emotional safety?
- Do their materials align with the statutory guidance and your school's approach to inclusivity?

We've worked hard to build trust and a supportive classroom environment, so it's crucial that any external input strengthens, rather than undermines, that culture.

Reflection Point

Take the time to consider the following:

- Have I reviewed the content and delivery style of any external PSHE providers we've used or are considering?
- How can I help ensure they support, not replace, the ongoing relationships and learning we've developed with our pupils?

Using guest speakers can be powerful, but they should be there to complement your teaching, not complicate it. With the right planning and debriefing, external input can spark conversations and deepen learning but only when it's grounded in the same thoughtful, pupil-centred approach that we aim for in every PSHE lesson.

The Role of Social Media and Popular Culture

We are now going to explore the role that social media and pop culture play in spreading myths and misconceptions about alcohol and drugs. It's not unusual for certain celebrities or influencers to glamorise drinking, getting drunk, taking drugs or getting high. This portrayal can be hugely misleading, especially for young people. They're often shown a version of someone's lifestyle that appears exciting, carefree and fun, but what they don't see is the reality behind the scenes. This person might be struggling with addiction, anxiety or depression. But that part of their life doesn't always make it onto their feed, at least not straight away, and often not at all.

The speed and reach of misinformation on platforms like TikTok, Snapchat, Instagram and YouTube are genuinely worrying. These apps are where many young people spend a large chunk of their time, and the information shared there can feel more real or relevant than what they hear in a lesson. When misinformation spreads so quickly, and when harmful behaviours are normalised or made to seem harmless or even aspirational, that's where the danger lies.

I've spoken about this in class. Pupils have watched a viral video where someone jokes about being drunk or high, and they assume it's just banter. But what they're not seeing are the long-term consequences that person might be facing. That's why this part of the education feels so important to me. It's about helping pupils understand what's real and what's not and giving them the tools to think critically about what they're seeing online.

On a personal level, I've always felt deeply about showing empathy towards people who are struggling, whether that's with addiction or their mental health. I've often heard young people use the term 'nitty' to describe people they assume are addicted to drugs. And honestly, it frustrates me.

Sometimes they'll see someone on the street who's clearly struggling, but without any understanding of that person's story, they'll just say, 'They are a nitty!' even when there's no evidence that person is using drugs.

That kind of thinking shows a lack of empathy, and it's something we need to challenge. I always say to my pupils, 'Instead of judging, ask yourself, how did that person get to this point? Who were they before this? What might they have gone through?' That kind of reflection helps young people examine their own assumptions and develop compassion for others. When we use derogatory labels to describe people with addiction, we run the risk of dehumanising people and reinforcing stigma around addiction and mental health. And I truly believe that's not ok. Teaching empathy and understanding must be central to our PSHE lessons because if we want to challenge stigma, we have to start with compassion.

The Role of Schools and Teachers in Harmful Substance Education

Let's now take a closer look at why it's so important that all teachers feel confident when it comes to teaching about harmful substances. There's a shared responsibility here, and it's not just down to PSHE leads to deliver this kind of content. Every teacher plays a part. Whether you're a subject teacher, a form tutor or part of the wider pastoral team, you have a role in reinforcing key messages and helping to create a safe space where pupils feel they can talk openly.

This toolkit is designed with that in mind. Even if you're not a specialist, you can still deliver this topic well and with confidence. That's one of the challenges many non-specialists face: not feeling qualified or unsure about how to approach the content. This is exactly why this book exists to give you the subject knowledge, the pedagogy and the tools to teach substance education with confidence and care.

Pupils are quick to pick up on a teacher's uncertainty or discomfort, and when they sense that, they're less likely to engage or speak up. Over the years, one of the biggest things I've learned is that when I feel confident and relaxed, the pupils respond in the same way. I'll be honest, when I first transitioned from leading PSHE in a primary setting for eight years to leading and teaching the subject in a secondary school, there were topics I just didn't want to teach. I avoided them. Pornography, STIs (sexually transmitted infections), FGM (female genital mutilation), it all felt so uncomfortable at the start. I skipped the lessons because I didn't have the confidence, I wasn't used to that age group and I didn't yet have the subject knowledge I needed.

But eventually, I had to face it. I realised that if I put myself in the shoes of the pupils and thought about how much they needed this information, it became harder to justify avoiding the subject. So I made a decision; I was going to teach it, and I was going to do it with as much confidence as I could find. And guess what? The more confident I felt, the more at ease the pupils were. Before long, it became completely natural to speak openly with them about difficult topics, and now I love teaching these parts of the curriculum.

One thing pupils really appreciate is honesty. If I don't know the answer to something, we find it out together. I don't pretend to know everything, and I don't need to. What matters more is empathy. Being able to put ourselves in their shoes and understand how they might be feeling when these topics come up. Some pupils will feel uncomfortable, and that's completely normal. That's why creating a safe classroom environment is so essential.

It's also important to think about the wider school community. Parents should be kept in the loop. I always advise informing them half-termly about what's being covered in PSHE. It helps to build trust and allows for open communication. At the same time, I make sure the pastoral team is fully aware of the topics we're covering and when. I usually send out a half-term staff email so that everyone is aware. This isn't just about being organised, it's about safeguarding. When staff know what's coming up in PSHE, they're better able to identify pupils who might need additional support or to keep an eye out for reactions to sensitive content.

Here are some organisations that could offer insights into strategies to use in the classroom and integrating harm reduction strategies:

- **The Drug Education Forum (DEF)**
  The DEF provides research and resources that outline best practices for delivering effective drug education in schools.

- **UK Government – Drug Strategy 2017**
  According to the HM Government (2017), this strategy tackles drug misuse, including educational interventions. It provides guidance for teachers and schools about the importance of an evidence-based approach to substance education.
- **FRANK – Substance Misuse Education**
  FRANK provides a detailed definitive listing of substances from A–Z, as well as advice and up-to-date news articles.

Strategies for Delivering Substance Education Effectively

One of the most important things to think about when teaching about harmful substances is how to create a safe and supportive space for learning. While some people refer to 'ground rules,' I prefer to call it a learner agreement. This isn't just something we impose on pupils, it's something we agree on together. It sets the tone for how we will speak and behave throughout the lesson. When we're talking about topics that can feel sensitive, emotional or even controversial, the teacher becomes a learner too. That shift helps build trust and shows pupils that we're in this together.

A great way to encourage honest dialogue is through anonymous questions. An anonymous question box is a brilliant tool to help pupils voice things they might feel too nervous to say out loud. I usually hand out Post-it notes, ask pupils to write their questions, fold them over and drop them into a box at the end of the session. At the start of the next lesson, I go through a selection of these and respond. It's a simple strategy, but it really empowers pupils to get the answers they need without drawing attention to themselves.

Using inclusive language can make all the difference in helping pupils feel seen, respected and safe to express themselves. It's also vital that we rely on evidence-based resources, not outdated scare tactics. Research from organisations like Mentor UK and the PSHE Association (2016) emphasises that scare-based approaches, such as 'Just Say No,' don't actually work. They may frighten some pupils, but they don't equip them with the tools they need to make informed decisions. Instead, we want pupils to be thoughtful, confident and well-informed, able to consider their values, understand the facts and make choices that support their well-being.

Lessons should include up-to-date information. Several studies shown on the NHS website remind us that substance trends evolve quickly. For example, vaping, cannabis edibles and nitrous oxide are far more prevalent now than a decade ago, and perceptions of risk have shifted. If we aren't using current, research-informed materials, we risk giving pupils advice that's no longer relevant, or worse, incorrect. Discussion-based learning is also key. I've found that when pupils are truly engaged, they often ask big, unexpected questions that lead us slightly off track. But these moments can be golden. I always try to follow their curiosity, as long as we stay grounded in the learning outcomes. Rather than giving a lecture, I encourage discussion. Using real-life scenarios can help pupils see how the decisions they make in the classroom might play out in real life. It turns theory into practice and gives them space to think critically.

It's also important to think about accessibility. When I'm planning for pupils with SEND or EAL, I use images to support new vocabulary and sometimes translate key words. Visual support and simple, clear explanations can go a long way in ensuring all pupils feel included.

Occasionally, a pupil might ask, 'Have you ever taken drugs?' It's a question that can catch teachers off guard. But it's essential to stay professional and keep boundaries in place. A response like this tends to work well:

> That's a really interesting question, and I can see why you might want to know more. But this lesson is about giving you the facts and tools to make informed choices, not about my personal life. What matters most is making sure you have accurate information and feel able to ask questions. Instead of focusing on people's personal stories, let's look at what we know from health experts, science and real-life data.

The reason this matters is because personal disclosures from staff can blur professional boundaries and create safeguarding risks. You're not there as a peer; you're there as a trusted adult. Maintaining that role helps pupils feel safe. Keeping the discussion focused on learning outcomes benefits everyone in the room.

Reflection Point

Take the time to consider the following:

- How do I create a safe, inclusive learning environment when delivering challenging topics like harmful substances?

Think about the strategies you currently use (e.g. learner agreements, inclusive language, differentiation and encouraging questions). Are there any areas where you could do more to make every pupil feel seen, heard and respected? What assumptions or habits might you need to challenge in yourself to better support open, honest and compassionate discussions?

Supporting Young People Beyond the Classroom

As teachers, we are in a unique position to notice when something isn't quite right. We see pupils regularly, often over a sustained period, and we become attuned to their baseline behaviours. When it comes to substance misuse, early identification can be a turning point. It's not about jumping to conclusions or labelling pupils, but also about being observant, reflective and responsive.

Identifying Signs of Substance Misuse

Substance misuse rarely exists in isolation. It is often linked with other vulnerabilities, including mental health struggles, adverse childhood experiences (ACEs) or peer pressure. Something that's come through clearly from young people is that they feel there aren't enough specialist services out there to support them when it comes to substance misuse (Public Health England, 2018). They want help that actually speaks to their experiences, and I think we really need to listen to that. Recognising the signs early can prevent escalation and ensure young people receive the support they need, when they first need it.

Signs of substance misuse can be physical, behavioural, emotional or social. These may include

- Red, bloodshot or glassy eyes.
- Unexplained weight changes.
- Frequent tiredness, lack of motivation or sudden bursts of energy.
- Smells of smoke or alcohol on breath or clothing.
- Significant mood swings, irritability or withdrawal.
- Sudden decline in academic performance.
- Changes in peer group or increased secrecy.
- Regularly missing school or leaving class without permission.

The most important sign is change. When a pupil who is usually punctual, enthusiastic and engaged starts showing up late, avoiding participation or withdrawing from social groups, it's worth pausing to reflect. Sometimes, these changes are subtle and unfold over time. Keeping a safeguarding log of these observations helps to build a fuller picture. We must approach this issue through a trauma-informed and non-judgemental lens. Substance use may be a coping mechanism, a response to distress or simply the result of peer influence. Young people don't need shame; they need support. According to the PSHE Association (2021), compassionate and consistent adult responses are vital in helping pupils feel safe enough to disclose concerns.

It's also important to understand the role of risk factors. Young people who experience instability at home, neglect, abuse or parental substance misuse are statistically more likely to experiment with harmful substances themselves (NHS Digital, 2023). However, these issues are not exclusive to any one demographic, and no pupil is immune, regardless of background.

How Teachers Can Provide Support and Intervention

Teachers are often the first trusted adults to notice when something isn't quite right. We might pick up on small changes: a pupil who's suddenly withdrawn or frequently tired or whose behaviour has shifted in subtle ways.

These aren't things to ignore. We're not expected to diagnose or investigate, but we are in a unique position to notice and respond with care.

The first step in providing meaningful support is knowing your role. You are not expected to be a counsellor, a therapist or a police officer. Your role is to be a consistent, calm adult who listens, observes and refers concerns through the appropriate channels. Sometimes that starts with a gentle conversation. Other times it means quietly logging your concerns and sharing them with your safeguarding lead. When a pupil does open up, it's vital we create space for them to be heard without fear of judgement. Letting a young person talk while staying calm and grounded, without reacting with shock or disapproval, can make all the difference. A helpful response might sound like: 'Thank you for trusting me with this. I'm really glad you've spoken to someone.' At that point, it's not about fixing the problem, but about making sure the right people are involved.

It's also important to follow safeguarding procedures correctly. Every school will have its own policy, but generally, if a pupil discloses substance misuse or you're concerned about their well-being, this must be recorded and passed on to the designated safeguarding lead (DSL). You may feel emotionally drawn in, especially if you know the pupil well, but the safest thing you can do is stick to your school's process. It ensures consistency, confidentiality and, above all, appropriate support.

Creating a culture of openness and care goes a long way. Pupils are far more likely to speak up if they feel safe and respected. This means that we should model respect, be consistent and show that we take all disclosures seriously. It also means maintaining boundaries. We are not their friends, but we can be trusted adults they turn to. The PSHE curriculum plays a big role in building this culture by creating regular opportunities for conversations around health, choices and well-being.

Remember, you don't need all the answers. What matters most is being present, staying grounded and making sure that the pupil doesn't feel like they're dealing with everything alone.

Engaging Parents and the Wider Community

Parents and carers are the first line of defence when it comes to preventing substance misuse among young people. They are often the first to notice subtle changes in behaviour, mood or social circles. Their influence is profound, and their involvement is crucial in both prevention and early intervention. One of the most effective ways parents can prevent substance misuse is by fostering open and honest relationships with their children. When young people feel they can talk to their parents without fear of judgement or punishment, they are more likely to share their experiences and concerns. According to YoungMinds (2024), normalising conversations about drugs and alcohol within the family can help children feel supported and informed, reducing the likelihood of risky behaviour. Parents serve as role models, and their attitudes and behaviours towards substances can significantly influence their children's choices. The NSPCC emphasises that while most parents use substances responsibly, those who misuse drugs or alcohol can struggle to meet their children's needs, potentially putting them at risk.

Understanding the challenges and pressures that young people face today is essential. Parents should stay informed about the substances their children might encounter and the associated risks. Engaging in their children's lives, including knowing their friends, interests and routines, can help parents detect early signs of trouble. Schools can play a pivotal role in supporting parents. Hosting workshops, providing informational materials and including helpful support sections in newsletters can equip parents with the tools they need to have meaningful conversations at home. Involving parents in educational initiatives can reinforce the messages delivered in the classroom, creating a consistent approach to substance education.

It's important for parents to know that they are not alone. Numerous organisations offer resources and support for families dealing with substance misuse:

- **FRANK**: Provides honest and confidential advice and information about drugs, their effects and the legal aspects.
- **We Are With You**: Offers free and confidential support for people with drug, alcohol or mental health problems, and their families.
- **Adfam**: A national charity working to campaign and support families affected by drugs and alcohol.
- **YoungMinds**: Provides support and guidance for parents on how to communicate with their children about drugs and alcohol.
- **NSPCC**: Offers support for parents who are worried about their own or someone else's substance use.

By leveraging these resources, parents can gain the knowledge and confidence needed to address substance misuse proactively.

Parents are integral to the prevention and early intervention of substance misuse among young people. Through open communication, positive role modelling, staying informed, collaborating with schools and accessing support services, they can create a protective and supportive environment that supports their child. Empowering parents with the right tools and knowledge is essential in safeguarding the well-being of their children.

What This Book Will Cover

This book is designed as a practical and supportive resource for teachers who are delivering education around harmful substances as part of their PSHE curriculum. It walks you through the process step by step, recognising that some teachers may feel unsure or lack confidence, especially if they are not PSHE specialists. It also acknowledges that even the most experienced teachers sometimes need new ideas, guidance or reassurance.

The next section of this book offers detailed teacher guidance. This section will focus on what you need to feel confident in your delivery. It begins with how to set up a safe learning environment, including how to create a learner agreement collaboratively with your pupils. You will find specific teaching tips that relate to the topic of harmful substances, including ways to recognise and respond to safeguarding concerns and disclosures. There is also a focus on using inclusive language and practices, so that every pupil feels seen and supported. The guidance will introduce the concept of using a normative approach, which helps pupils to understand that not everyone engages in risky behaviours. You will also find advice on working with external providers, assessment approaches that fit PSHE and suggestions on how to keep parents and carers informed. This section ends with ideas for making cross-topic and cross-curricular links, helping to embed harmful substance education more deeply across the school experience.

Following the teacher guidance section are 18 full lesson plans, divided across the three Key Stages, along with 18 tutor time plans. These are also divided equally across Key Stage 3, Key Stage 4 and Key Stage 5. The tutor time sessions are designed to be used by form tutors or non-specialists and are deliberately kept light. They are a great way to consolidate learning from the main lessons, give pupils time to reflect, revisit key messages and develop their thinking and values. The tutor time plans do not include sensitive content and are an opportunity to revisit key skills and knowledge in a calm, consistent way. They work particularly well as conversation starters and gentle prompts for pupils to remember what they learned.

Each lesson in this book is carefully structured to last around 50 minutes and is designed to offer both clarity and flexibility. The format follows a consistent, supportive rhythm: a brief **starter activity** to spark engagement and curiosity, followed by a **main activity** that delves into the key theme. This is then rounded off with a short **wrap-up or assessment moment**, giving pupils a chance to reflect or consolidate their learning. Each lesson also ends with a **signposting and teacher confidence section**, offering teachers an opportunity to give pupils guidance on where they can seek further help, information or support, which is a crucial step in building awareness and promoting well-being.

Rather than framing topics in rigid binaries like 'healthy versus unhealthy,' these lessons encourage **open discussion**, **critical thinking** and **personal reflection**. The emphasis is on creating a space where young people can explore ideas safely and honestly and where diverse perspectives are welcomed.

Wherever specific resources are needed to deliver an activity, they are clearly highlighted within the lesson plans. These may include printed worksheets, scenario cards, case studies or debate planners. Each resource is labelled (e.g. 'KS4 Lesson 3 Resource 1') to make preparation and delivery as straightforward as possible without needing to reinvent the wheel. While the core structure provides a clear path, there's also **room for adaptation**, allowing you to tailor activities to your setting or the needs of your pupils, without losing the heart of the message. Ultimately, these lessons are about connection, empowerment and equipping young people with the tools to think for themselves and make informed, confident choices.

This book is designed with both specialist and non-specialist teachers in mind, recognising that delivering education about harmful substances can feel daunting. To help you approach this important topic confidently, the guidance offers clear explanations of key concepts without jargon, making the subject accessible regardless of your prior knowledge. Each lesson plan provides a step-by-step structure, carefully guiding you through activities and discussions. This approach saves you valuable time on planning and ensures you have the tools to deliver lessons effectively and sensitively. Understanding that some topics may be sensitive or raise questions beyond your expertise, the book also includes advice on managing classroom conversations and responding to disclosures with care and professionalism. Where needed, it signposts external organisations and specialist professionals who can offer further support, helping you to know when and how to seek additional help. Practical tips on creating an inclusive and safe learning environment are woven throughout, ensuring all pupils feel supported and respected.

Ultimately, this resource is a toolkit that equips you to deliver confident, informed and meaningful education about harmful substances. It empowers you to focus on what matters most, which in turn helps your pupils stay safe, informed and empowered. The power to teach this important content lies within you. Believe in yourself and have confidence in your ability to make a real difference. Sometimes nerves and self-doubt can creep in but remember the simple phrase that has helped me through many moments . . . *Just Do It*. Our young people need to learn these topics, and it is our duty to teach them with passion and commitment.

How to Use This Book

This book is designed to be practical, supportive and flexible. Think of it as a toolkit: something you can dip in and out of, adapt for your setting and use in a way that feels right for you and your pupils.

Each lesson plan follows a clear and consistent structure to make planning as straightforward as possible. You'll find

- Lesson titles and pupil-friendly objectives.
- Key vocabulary and resources.
- A structured flow.
- Assessment ideas built into the session.
- Signposting to support services relevant to each topic.
- Teacher tips and confidence boosts to guide delivery.

Each lesson has a clear starter, main activity and plenary. Assessment ideas are built into every stage to help you track progress and respond to pupils' needs in real time. Read the whole plan before teaching so you can prepare for all of the assessment ideas from the very start of the lesson.

You'll also find suggested tutor time activities for each Key Stage after the lesson plan section. These can be used as standalone sessions or as lighter-touch follow-ups to reinforce the learning. If you're tight on time, nervous about the topic or just not sure where to begin, starting with these short activities can be a great way in.

If you're new to teaching about substances, or just feeling unsure, please know: you don't need to be an expert. This book is here to help you feel prepared, not perfect. The lessons are written to be accessible, supportive and safe, for both you and your pupils. Take your time, adapt what you need and don't be afraid to go slowly or split a lesson across more than one session. What matters most is that pupils feel safe, heard and well-informed.

2 Teacher Guidance

This chapter is designed to support you in delivering substance education with confidence, care and clarity, whether you're a PSHE specialist or not. It offers practical strategies, safeguarding advice and inclusive teaching approaches that reflect the reality of working with diverse pupils in today's classrooms. You don't need to be an expert in drugs or alcohol to use this guidance. You just need to be willing to create a safe space for pupils to explore, reflect and learn. This isn't about delivering perfect lessons. It's about feeling prepared, supported and equipped to make a real difference.

When we talk about substance education, it's easy to assume it only happens within the PSHE classroom or is the responsibility of a specialist teacher. But the reality is, all teachers play a vital role in this area. Safeguarding means that every teacher, regardless of subject, has a duty to help keep children safe and that includes recognising the risks around substance use and misuse. The Department for Education's statutory guidance, *Keeping Children Safe in Education* (2024), emphasises this by stating that the 'safeguarding and promoting the welfare of children is everyone's responsibility.' The guidance also mentions that the use of alcohol and drugs may also be a sign of child sexual exploitation.

We need to acknowledge the fact that PSHE is often taught by non-specialists who may have been asked to deliver lessons on harmful substances without any 'high quality training and support' (Department for Education & Association of Chief Police Officers, 2012). This can be daunting but that is what makes this guidance so important. Whether you are a form tutor, a subject teacher or part of the wider pastoral team, you have a significant role to play. Simply knowing how

DOI: 10.4324/9781003608998-2

to spot concerns early on, being confident in your subject knowledge and being open to having honest conversations with pupils can make a real difference.

Tutor time is a brilliant opportunity to build meaningful relationships with pupils. That consistent daily or weekly contact helps to create a sense of safety and trust. These interactions might seem small, but they go a long way. Pupils are more likely to open up to someone they feel knows them, respects them and listens to them without judgement. Teachers have more influence than they often realise. By modelling healthy behaviours, setting clear expectations and creating space for open dialogue, we help to shape how young people think about substances. Even informal chats in corridors, classrooms or during after-school clubs all contribute to the culture we create. So it's not just about delivering a lesson, it's also about recognising the quiet, powerful ways in which we support and protect our pupils every day.

Whole-School Culture and Messaging

The Department for Education and the Association of Chief Police Officers 'Drug Advice for Schools' report (2012) highlights that harmful substance education is most useful when 'supported by the whole school community.' When we talk about building a whole-school culture around harmful substance education, we are not just talking about what happens in the PSHE lessons. It includes a wider ethos that is felt in the corridors, in conversations and in the choices made at all levels of the school. It's about making sure that every member of staff is informed, confident and ready to reinforce consistent messages that help young people stay safe and make responsible decisions.

A healthy school culture in this area starts with education. Staff need to feel confident, not only in their subject knowledge but also in the language they use when discussing sensitive topics like drug or alcohol use. We must approach this in a way that is non-judgemental and rooted in safeguarding. When a pupil discloses a concern or a teacher notices a worrying pattern of behaviour, the reaction must be calm, informed and focused on support. A strong culture is one where pupils feel safe to open up, knowing they will be met with compassion rather than punishment or shame. It's also important that school policies reflect current trends, research and best practice.

They need to be living documents, reviewed regularly, shaped by the latest data and clearly communicated to staff. If we are working with outdated approaches or vague guidelines, we risk leaving pupils vulnerable and staff uncertain of what to do when situations occur. The language we use also matters too. We want to avoid an 'anti-substance' tone that can shut down conversations. Instead, we should frame our approach as pro-health and pro-safety, helping pupils to understand the risks and make better choices without feeling judged.

This culture should be visible in school life. This could include well-thought-out assemblies and the use of credible and relevant external agencies; even displays in the corridors can play a part. Pastoral teams, in particular, can take the lead in sharing trends and updates and still ensure that there is no breach of confidentiality. There's a lot of valuable information that can be cascaded to help staff respond proactively. It's a small shift that could make a big impact. As mentioned previously, tutor time is a key space where relationships are built and trust is developed. This isn't something for us to underestimate. It's often in those informal moments that real connection and influence can happen. When teachers use that time intentionally to reinforce positive behaviours and open up conversation, we become powerful role models. This is where culture is really built, in the daily, authentic interactions between staff and pupils.

Framing Within Safeguarding and Well-being

Teaching about harmful substances cannot be separated from a school's safeguarding responsibilities. According to the 'Keeping Children Safe in Education' (DfE, 2024) statutory guidance, 'drug taking and/or alcohol misuse may be signs that children are at risk.' This means that substance education is not simply about informing pupils of risks, but also about identifying when they might be vulnerable, at risk of harm or in need of early intervention. As teachers, we have a duty to be vigilant and to take seriously any signs of substance misuse, but this needs to be balanced with compassion and an understanding of the whole child. Taboos surrounding drug and alcohol misuse may lead to stigmatising views, and when punitive or judgemental attitudes are present in school cultures, this can reinforce harmful notions of 'right' versus 'wrong' behaviour (Waples et al., 2023). Instead of fear-based approaches, we need to build a climate of care where pupils feel safe enough to speak up and ask for help.

A more supportive approach might look like explicitly teaching well-being strategies, helping pupils understand how to maintain good mental and physical health and, most importantly, fostering self-worth and resilience. Loving oneself and feeling valued can make a significant difference in the choices young people make. When education around substances is delivered in this context of support, it can become transformative. Teachers also play an essential role in signposting pupils to professional support when needed. It is not about having all the answers, but about being a trusted adult who listens, responds without judgement and helps pupils to get the help they deserve.

Reflection Point

Think about how substance use has been framed in your school so far.

- Have there been opportunities for open, non-judgemental conversations?
- What could you do in your role, no matter your subject or position, to contribute to a more supportive, safeguarding-led culture when teaching or discussing harmful substances?

Why All Non-Specialist Teachers Need Confidence

One of the most common barriers to teaching about harmful substances is the belief that you need to be an expert. I've heard so many teachers say, 'I wouldn't know where to begin,' or 'I'm not qualified to talk about drugs.' I understand that these topics can feel sensitive, daunting or even personal. Sometimes a lack of subject knowledge can make teachers feel out of their depth. But the truth is, you don't need to know everything. What matters most is being open, prepared and willing to learn alongside your pupils.

It's also important to acknowledge that personal experience plays a role in shaping how confident teachers feel. Some staff may have lived through difficult situations themselves or with people close to them, and that can make the subject feel too close for comfort. Others may worry about saying the wrong thing or being asked something they can't answer. These are natural concerns, but they shouldn't stop us from doing this important work. With the right support, any teacher can grow into this role.

Another myth I've come across is the idea that talking about drugs or alcohol might 'put ideas' into pupils' heads, but open, honest conversations about harmful substances, when done well, can help young people to make informed decisions and feel more confident navigating real-life situations. Silence, on the other hand, can leave gaps that misinformation or peer pressure quickly fill. Confidence grows through practice, good training and a supportive school culture. Whether you've been teaching PSHE for years or you're just stepping into it, your presence and care make a difference. The most powerful thing you can bring to the classroom isn't expertise. It's empathy, consistency and a willingness to show up.

The 'Non-Speci-alist' Teacher and Their Power

To be completely frank, most of what makes substance education impactful isn't about reciting facts. It's about the way those facts are delivered. Non-specialist teachers often already use dynamic, pupil-led approaches in their own subjects. They're familiar with questioning techniques, active learning, scaffolding ideas and building rapport. These skills are crucial when delivering sensitive or potentially challenging content. A well-planned, interactive session delivered with confidence can be far more effective than a flat, one-way delivery from a so-called 'expert.'

In many ways, being a non-specialist is a hidden advantage. You are learning alongside your pupils, modelling curiosity, openness and humility. If a question comes up and you don't know the answer, that's okay. This is an excellent opportunity to explore the answer together. What you do need is the confidence to hold space for real conversation and the skills to guide pupils in thinking critically and making informed choices.

There's also something quite powerful in being honest about your own learning. Pupils can sense when a teacher is genuinely engaged. If you say, 'This isn't my area of expertise, but I've done my research and we're going to work through this together,' you're showing that learning is a shared process. You're reinforcing that this topic matters, no matter what subject you usually teach.

We also have to challenge the myth that only certain staff can 'handle' PSHE topics. Every teacher has the ability to help pupils reflect on their health, safety and well-being. Every teacher can create a safe and open space. And every teacher, regardless of their subject or role, has the capacity to positively shape attitudes and behaviours.

So if you're a non-specialist, please know this: YOU ARE ENOUGH! With the right guidance and tools, you can teach about harmful substances in a way that is meaningful and memorable. This toolkit exists to support you with that. It is here to help you build your confidence, back up your teaching with sound pedagogy and remind you that your presence in the classroom matters. You don't need to be perfect. You just need to show up, stay open and keep learning . . . just like your pupils.

Building Trust With Pupils Through Presence

Building trust in the classroom is foundational to teaching about harmful substances. Pupils are far more likely to engage in meaningful discussions, ask honest questions and reflect deeply when they feel safe, respected and understood. One of the most effective ways to establish this trust is through the consistent presence and approach of the teacher, not just physically, but emotionally and relationally too.

One of the first things I do at the start of a scheme of work is establish a learner agreement with the class. Some might call this 'ground rules,' but I've always found 'agreement' better reflects the collaborative nature of it. This is something we create together, where pupils actively contribute ideas on how we will treat each other and behave during lessons that may cover sensitive topics. This helps set a tone of mutual respect and shared responsibility. It not only gives pupils a voice, but it also reminds them that their voice matters.

Humour can also play a big part. When used appropriately, it has a disarming quality and helps pupils feel relaxed and comfortable. Being open and honest with pupils is another powerful way to strengthen rapport. Of course, this doesn't mean sharing personal details but rather being transparent about your role. I make it clear that the classroom is a private and safe space for discussion, but I also gently explain the safeguarding responsibilities I have. I explain that if I'm ever concerned that a pupil is at risk, I have to pass that on to ensure they get the right support. Being upfront about this from the start builds a sense of emotional safety while establishing trust in your role as a protective adult.

Small actions matter too. Even something as simple as closing the classroom door, if there is a window, at the start of a session can subtly signal that this space is now 'ours.' It is important to create a respectful environment where open dialogue is welcome. Checking in with pupils individually, noticing shifts in their mood or behaviour and being consistent in your reactions all contribute to how safe a pupil feels in your presence.

Ultimately, presence is about being human with your pupils. We can do this by showing empathy, warmth and genuine interest in their well-being. Trust is built lesson by lesson, moment by moment and when pupils feel that from their teacher, particularly in PSHE, the impact can be long-lasting. It means they're more likely to speak up when something is wrong, ask the question that's on their mind and walk away from a lesson feeling seen, heard and better equipped to make healthy, informed decisions.

Safeguarding Responsibilities and Recognising Risk Factors

Spotting the signs of substance use or misuse in young people can be difficult, especially when you consider how subtle or ambiguous some indicators might be. According to the UK Addiction Treatment Centres, signs might include red or watery eyes, changes in mood or personality, truancy, memory problems or shifts in friendship groups. You might also notice a decline in academic performance or differences in hygiene and appearance. But here's the important part! No single sign automatically points to substance use. Teachers must be cautious not to make assumptions. For example, red eyes might be caused by hay fever. Changes in behaviour might relate to mental health, family issues or neurodivergence. That's why it's vital for staff to receive proper training not just in what to look for but also in how to interpret potential indicators within the broader context of each pupil's life.

We have to trust our professional intuition but not rely on guesswork. The goal isn't to diagnose or label, it's to remain alert, aware and supportive. Being trauma-informed means understanding that behaviours often communicate a need, not just a problem. That subtle shift in perspective allows us to be more compassionate and proactive rather than punitive or judgemental. Creating a culture where staff feel confident sharing concerns and are clear on reporting procedures is just as important as knowing the signs themselves. Often, teachers fear saying the wrong thing or overreacting. However, when we have systems in place, like designated safeguarding leads and clear referral pathways, that fear can be replaced with clarity and action.

Safeguarding is everyone's responsibility and that includes being attentive to risk factors like potential substance misuse. It's not just the job of the PSHE teacher. Every member of staff who interacts with young people has a part to play in noticing when something isn't quite right, keeping an open mind and following safeguarding procedures to make sure the right support can be offered early.

Handling Disclosures Safely

When a pupil chooses to disclose something sensitive, especially relating to substance use or harm, it's a significant moment that requires a careful and compassionate response. As teachers, our immediate priority should be to listen attentively and ensure the pupil feels heard and supported. In the moment of a disclosure, the most important thing a teacher can do is create a calm, safe space where the pupil feels genuinely heard and supported. Pupils should be allowed to speak at their own pace, without being interrupted or steered by leading questions. Simply listening can go a long way. It's vital to acknowledge their courage in opening up and let them know they have done the right thing by speaking to you. At the same time, it's essential to be clear and honest about what will happen next. This includes explaining that you may need to pass the information on to the safeguarding team, not as a punishment, but to help protect their safety and well-being. Being transparent helps to build trust and shows that safeguarding is about care, not control.

According to the Department for Education's guidance, 'Keeping Children Safe in Education' (2024), all staff should be aware of the procedures for handling disclosures and must report any concerns about a child's welfare immediately to the designated safeguarding lead (DSL) or a deputy. After the disclosure, make a clear and factual record of what was said, using the pupil's own words as much as possible. Note the date, time and any observations about the pupil's demeanour. This record should be passed on promptly to the DSL, who will determine the appropriate course of action, which may involve contacting external agencies.

It's crucial to remember that our role is not to investigate but to report concerns to the appropriate safeguarding personnel. Maintaining confidentiality is important, but it should never come at the expense of a child's safety. Always follow your school's safeguarding policies and procedures and seek guidance from the DSL if you're unsure about any aspect of handling a disclosure. By responding to disclosures with empathy, honesty and adherence to safeguarding protocols, we can ensure that pupils receive the support they need while upholding our duty of care.

Escalation Routes and Staff Duties Under 'Keeping Children Safe in Education'

All teachers, regardless of their subject specialism, have a statutory duty to safeguard children. This includes recognising and escalating concerns related to potential substance misuse. Under 'Keeping Children Safe in Education' (KCSIE) (DfE, 2024), any sign that a pupil may be misusing drugs or alcohol, or is at risk of doing so, must be taken seriously and reported appropriately. It's vital that teachers feel confident in what to do next. While the DSL will take forward any investigation or response, the role of the classroom teacher is to spot potential indicators and report them clearly and promptly.

Here are some key responsibilities all staff should keep in mind:

- **Know the safeguarding policy**: Every school will have its own child protection policy. Familiarising yourself with it ensures that you know who to go to and how to report concerns.
- **Follow escalation procedures**: Concerns should be passed to the DSL immediately. If the DSL is unavailable, the deputy DSL or a senior leader should be approached without delay.
- **Report factually and professionally**: When reporting a concern, be clear and specific. Stick to the facts: what you saw, heard or noticed. Avoid including your personal opinions or assumptions.
- **Use the correct systems**: Most schools now use digital safeguarding reporting tools. Make sure you are comfortable using these, and if in doubt, ask for training or guidance.
- **Do not promise confidentiality**: It's crucial that pupils understand that if they disclose something that puts them or others at risk, you must pass this information on to keep them safe.
- **Be mindful of bias**: Avoid making assumptions based on appearance, background or behaviour. A non-judgemental, trauma-informed approach helps maintain trust and professionalism.

Raising concerns is not about making a diagnosis or handling a situation alone, it is about playing your part in a wider system of care. Teachers often worry they'll say the wrong thing or overreact, but the real risk is in saying nothing at all.

Inclusion, Representation and Trauma-Informed Practice

Representation matters deeply when educating young people about harmful substances. When pupils can see aspects of their identity reflected in the curriculum, they are more likely to feel included and respected, and that contributes to more effective and meaningful learning.

In my own practice, I am very intentional about the imagery and case studies that I use. For example, I make sure to include people from different cultures and ethnicities in the visuals within lesson slides. This is particularly important in the context of substance education, as there are harmful stereotypes about what a 'typical' drug user or dealer looks like. Substance misuse affects individuals from all racial and cultural backgrounds, and our materials must reflect that reality rather than reinforce narrow or prejudicial assumptions. When writing scenarios or case studies, I often use unisex names and neutral 'they' pronouns so that pupils are not making unconscious assumptions about gender. This approach helps avoid assigning stereotypical roles and allows more pupils to relate to the characters. I also think it's important to represent a variety of family structures. I might include characters from same-sex families or use examples of single fathers to gently challenge norms and broaden pupils' understanding of different lived experiences.

These decisions may seem small, but they have a powerful impact. If pupils don't see themselves represented or if they only ever see certain groups portrayed negatively, it can reinforce harmful biases. As teachers, we must actively work to ensure the curriculum doesn't just educate, but also affirms identity, challenges prejudice and opens up safe space for dialogue.

Trauma-Informed Delivery Principles

Creating a safe, inclusive and emotionally supportive learning environment is at the heart of effective substance education. It can't be said enough. Teaching about potentially triggering topics like drug or alcohol misuse requires more than subject knowledge; it calls for sensitivity, compassion and awareness of pupils' emotional needs. A trauma-informed approach supports pupils who may be carrying lived experience or trauma related to substance misuse, either personally or through someone close to them. One of the most powerful tools in setting the tone for this type of learning is the teacher/learner agreement. Starting the session with a clear, collaboratively agreed set of expectations helps to create emotional safety. It sets out what is expected of everyone in the room, including the teacher. This agreement can be revisited during the lesson when needed to reinforce a consistent message: the classroom is a respectful and safe space for learning and reflection.

Positioning yourself as a learner alongside your pupils can also help build trust and break down perceived barriers. When pupils see that you are open to learning and that you don't have all the answers, it humanises the interaction. It encourages them to engage without fear of judgement. Before beginning a lesson on a sensitive topic, I always provide pupils with a heads-up the week before. This gives them time to process, seek support if needed or make me aware if they might find the content difficult. Some pupils may want to speak to you in private after the session, and offering this space in advance can make a big difference.

In my classroom, I keep an anonymous box where pupils can leave notes, questions or concerns. At the start of the next session, I respond to these contributions in a thoughtful and supportive way. This allows pupils to engage with the topic even if they don't feel comfortable speaking out loud. It also gives me insight into what they are thinking or feeling without putting them on the spot. Journals are another helpful strategy. Pupils can use these to reflect, ask questions or express their thoughts during the session. The journals aren't marked or assessed, and pupils are reminded that they won't be judged on what they write. However, I make it clear from the beginning that I will read the journals to ensure pupil safety and to fulfil my safeguarding responsibilities. While they are not a private diary, they provide an important space for quieter voices to be heard and for disclosures to be made in a way that feels safe.

Overall, being trauma-informed is about anticipating that some pupils will come into the room carrying difficult experiences and then teaching in a way that doesn't compound harm. It's about consistency, care and creating a climate where pupils feel protected, seen and heard.

Inclusion for SEND and EAL Learners

The PSHE Association (2025) offers practical and thoughtful guidance in their resource 'Teaching Pupils With SEND About Alcohol and Other Drugs.' They rightly point out that 'key vocabulary' can be 'listed on each lesson plan but you may choose to use additional visual or symbolic images to support pupils' understanding.' This might include using widget images to support written content or offering physical objects instead of pictures for pupils who learn more effectively through touch. For some, projecting a resource onto a screen rather than handing out a paper copy might make all the difference. In my own experience, I've found that these small adjustments often go a long way. Pupils with additional needs tend to respond much better when resources are tailored to their learning styles and preferences. It's not about rewriting everything. We can make small, thoughtful changes that can transform the way a pupil engages. Throughout the lesson plans included in this book, I've made a conscious effort to embed inclusive strategies that support learners with SEND without singling them out. The approach has been about flexibility, clarity and accessibility, making sure that all pupils can engage meaningfully, no matter their starting point.

Key adaptations include breaking learning down into manageable steps, using visual aids where appropriate and offering multiple ways for pupils to participate, whether that's through discussion, paired tasks or short written reflections. I've incorporated clear signposting and key vocabulary checks in each lesson plan, which help to support understanding and reduce cognitive overload. Wherever possible, tasks are scaffolded and instructions are given verbally and visually to suit different processing needs. The lesson plans also include low-stakes, confidence-building activities early in lessons so learners can feel successful from the outset. Group roles and flexible seating can help reduce anxiety and allow pupils to work in a way that suits them best. Finally, I've kept in mind that not all learners will be comfortable contributing in large groups, so there are opportunities for private reflection or smaller pair work instead. The goal has been to create lessons that feel safe, structured and supportive for everyone, especially those who need that extra bit of scaffolding to thrive.

For pupils who are new to the English language, especially those who have recently arrived at our school, I provide resources and worksheets in their home language wherever possible. This ensures that the learning is genuinely accessible and helps those pupils feel like they truly belong in the classroom. This sense of inclusion is essential, particularly when exploring a topic as sensitive and personal as harmful substances. These kinds of adaptations don't just benefit individual pupils. They can help the whole classroom. Strategies like visual scaffolding, simplified instructions, key vocabulary banks and structured lesson flow can help everyone focus, follow and reflect. Inclusion isn't just for our SEND and EAL pupils; it's part of good teaching.

Most importantly, teachers should feel empowered to adapt lessons as needed. It's this kind of flexibility and responsiveness that helps all pupils feel seen, supported and able to engage with the learning on their own terms.

Avoiding Shame and Bias

When teaching about drugs and alcohol, we have to be mindful of the way our own views and experiences may influence how we present the topic. Sometimes, without realising it, teachers can express judgements or assumptions that may be rooted in personal beliefs or societal stereotypes. This can come across in the way we speak during a lesson, the tone we use or even in the language in our resources. For pupils who may have lived experience of substance use, either personally or through a family member, this can unintentionally cause shame or guilt. That's never our goal in PSHE education.

A key part of delivering substance education responsibly is creating a space where all pupils feel safe, respected and not judged. This means avoiding framing drug or alcohol use as purely a matter of right and wrong. Instead, we can focus on the health implications, informed decision-making and the importance of knowing how and where to get help. The aim is to equip pupils with the knowledge and tools they need, not to shame or frighten them into compliance. As teachers, we also need to be aware that the young people in our classroom may already hold biased or stigmatising views towards those who use substances. Our teaching should actively challenge these ideas and help pupils think critically. For example, we can avoid language that labels people with addiction and dehumanises them and instead talk about people living with substance dependency or those affected by it. It's about modelling compassionate and respectful dialogue.

As mentioned previously, using inclusive and diverse resources also helps. Case studies that show a wide range of backgrounds, family setups and lived experiences make it clear that substance use does not affect just one type of person. When we include a variety of voices and perspectives, we help pupils understand that this is a complex issue, and everyone deserves support and understanding and not judgement. Our responsibility is not just to teach facts. It is to shape values and behaviours. This all starts with how we approach the subject ourselves.

Parental Engagement and Keeping Families Informed

The DfE's statutory guidance on 'Relationships Education, Relationships and Sex Education (RSE) and Health Education' reminds us that 'parents and carers are the prime teachers for children on many of these matters.' This is especially true when it comes to sensitive topics like drugs and alcohol. Rather than working in isolation, schools should approach substance education as a shared responsibility. That means creating opportunities for open and honest communication with parents that is clear, regular and thoughtful. Good communication can make all the difference. When parents understand what their children are learning, they feel more confident continuing those conversations at home. The RSE and Health Education guidance encourages schools to show parents the resources being used in class, as this can offer reassurance and help build trust. In my own practice, I've found that this small step can significantly ease parent anxiety and foster more supportive home environments.

One simple but effective method is through half-term newsletters. These can outline the topics being covered in PSHE and offer tips or questions for parents to explore at home. Another useful approach is parent workshops. These allow for more interactive discussion, helping to build understanding and provide clarity around the language and approach being used. It also gives parents the chance to ask questions and feel part of the learning journey. It is best to avoid a one-sided relationship where schools inform and parents receive. Instead, this should feel like a partnership, one where everyone is working together in the best interest of the child.

Reducing Stigma and Building Trust

Reducing the stigma around substance use is one of the most powerful and necessary steps schools can take in building trust with pupils and families. Stigma often acts as a barrier to openness, to seeking help and to accessing support. In schools, we have the opportunity to challenge unhelpful narratives and reshape the language and attitudes that surround this topic. Too often, stigma is reinforced unintentionally through the language we hear in everyday conversations. Many parents may still refer to individuals experiencing substance misuse using outdated or harmful labels such as 'junkie,' 'pothead' or 'alcoholic.' These words can carry significant shame and make it harder for young people to view substance use as a health issue rather than a moral failing. According to the National Institute on Drug Abuse (2021), stigmatising language can prevent individuals, including children and young people, from seeking treatment. This is a key reason why it is so important that teachers lead the way by modelling compassionate, person-first language.

When talking about substance use in the classroom, terms such as 'person with a substance use disorder' or 'person who misuses alcohol' are preferred. These alternatives remove blame or character judgement and allow pupils to engage with the content without fear of being judged or alienated. Using these terms also sends a clear message that the classroom is a safe, respectful space where the teacher recognises that there are complex social, emotional and health-related factors behind substance use. Establishing a culture of trust takes time but begins with consistency. Being mindful of our own biases and avoiding assumptions about pupils' home lives, backgrounds or personal choices contributes to a more inclusive environment. Using case studies that challenge stereotypes and giving pupils the tools to critically analyse what they hear at home, online or in wider society can also help to dismantle shame.

Finally, building trust is not just about how we teach but how we respond. If a pupil discloses something personal, how we listen, react and follow up can either reinforce or break their sense of safety. We cannot underestimate the value of being calm, non-judgemental and open. Trust is the foundation for meaningful learning, and it is our responsibility to build it during the discussions in our lessons.

Involving Parents in Preventative Education

When it comes to preventing substance misuse, parents are not just supporters, they are partners in the educational journey. Schools must move beyond simply informing parents and instead work to empower them with the tools, language and confidence to engage in preventative education at home. One of the most powerful ways to do this is by helping parents understand their influence. The Substance Abuse and Mental Health Services Administration (SAMHSA) emphasises that parents have a significant influence on their children's decisions regarding alcohol and drug use. Their guidance states,

> When parents create supportive and nurturing environments, children make better decisions. Though it may not always seem like it, children really hear their parents' concerns, which is why it's important that parents discuss the risks of using alcohol and other drugs.

We need to support parents in knowing when and how to have these conversations, not only during moments of crisis, but also as part of normal, everyday family life. Workshops and parent information evenings can be a helpful way to share practical strategies and answer difficult questions. These events are also opportunities to challenge myths, reduce stigma and break down any taboos parents may hold around drugs and alcohol. In some cases, providing guidance on how to talk to teens without judgement or fear can be incredibly powerful.

Schools can also make resources accessible at home, such as conversation starters, videos or key vocabulary lists, to help parents feel included and not overwhelmed. The aim is not to turn parents into experts, but to support them in their vital role as the first line of prevention. By inviting parents into this space with empathy and clarity, we make substance education more meaningful, consistent and effective for every pupil.

Working With External Agencies and Guest Speakers

One of the most important decisions when bringing in external agencies or guest speakers is to ensure they are both effective and safe contributors. It's not just about filling a slot in the timetable or getting someone else to teach about a difficult topic, it's about enhancing pupils' learning and supporting them in a way that feels relevant, trustworthy and consistent with your school's values. An effective contributor goes beyond simply sharing facts about harmful substances. They have up-to-date, evidence-based knowledge that reflects current research and local realities. This helps ensure pupils receive accurate information rather than myths or scare stories. For example, referencing trusted sources like NHS Digital or Public Health England can make discussions feel credible and grounded in real data.

Relatability plays a huge role in effectiveness. Pupils are more likely to engage when the speaker connects with their experiences, speaks in a natural, age-appropriate way and shows empathy without judgement. Talking about substances can be sensitive and sometimes triggering, so it's vital that contributors create a calm, supportive space where pupils feel safe to listen, ask questions and reflect.

Delivery style is just as important. The most impactful visitors use interactive methods such as discussions, role-plays or scenarios, encouraging pupils to think critically and participate actively. This approach fosters deeper understanding and helps pupils explore their own values and choices.

Above all, any external contributor must align with your school's policies, curriculum and ethos. This alignment supports a coherent learning journey and reinforces the messages pupils hear in the classroom. To ensure this, ask yourself the following:

- Are you clear about the aims and objectives the external contributor plans to deliver?
- Does their session complement, rather than replace, teacher-led activities?
- Do you understand the learning outcomes they aim to achieve?
- Have they been properly vetted according to your school's safeguarding procedures?
- Are you confident they understand and will follow safeguarding protocols, including how to handle disclosures?
- How will the contributor be supervised during the session to ensure pupil safety?
- Have pupils been prepared for the session, and will there be an opportunity to debrief afterwards?

By carefully considering these questions and working collaboratively with contributors, schools can bring valuable expertise into the classroom without compromising safety or consistency. This partnership enriches substance education and ensures it remains meaningful and supportive for every pupil.

Preparing and Debriefing With Pupils

Bringing an external contributor into your classroom can be a powerful way to enrich substance education, but it's important to prepare pupils beforehand and debrief with them afterwards. These steps help create a safe and supportive learning environment, where pupils know what to expect and can process what they've learned thoughtfully. Preparation begins by setting clear expectations. Before the session, explain who the visitor is and why they're coming. This helps reduce any anxiety and builds trust. You might say something like, 'Next week, we'll have a guest speaker who works with young people around substance use. They're here to share facts, answer your questions and support you to make informed choices.' Make sure pupils know that the session is a safe space where their questions and feelings are respected.

It can also be helpful to establish or revisit your classroom learning agreement at this point, reminding pupils about confidentiality, respect and listening without judgement. You could introduce an anonymous question box to give pupils a way to ask questions they might feel uncomfortable raising aloud. This encourages openness while protecting privacy.

After the session, debriefing is just as crucial. You should provide time for pupils to reflect on what they've learned and to express any thoughts or concerns. This can be done through group discussion, written reflection or paired conversations. The goal is to help pupils process information, clarify any misunderstandings and connect the learning to their own lives. During debriefs, be attentive to any safeguarding concerns that might arise. Some pupils may disclose personal experiences or emotions triggered by the session. Be ready to listen calmly, follow your school's safeguarding protocols and reassure pupils that support is available. From my experience, it's also useful to have a seating plan prepared with pupils' names.

Sometimes, external contributors may approach you after a session to share information about a pupil or show a piece of writing or drawing, but if they don't know the pupil's name or who sat where, this can create a safeguarding risk. Without that vital detail, there's a missed opportunity to provide timely support to a young person who might be silently asking for help. Having a seating plan on hand ensures you can respond quickly and appropriately, keeping pupils safe and supported.

Finally, link the visitor's session back to your ongoing teaching. Reinforce key messages, revisit important facts and explore any themes that came up. This helps embed learning and shows that substance education is a continuous conversation, not a one-off event. By carefully preparing and debriefing pupils, you maximise the impact of external contributions and create a safe, respectful space where young people feel empowered to engage and learn.

Aligning With Curriculum, Not Replacing It

External contributors can offer valuable expertise and fresh perspectives in substance education. However, their role must always be to complement the school's curriculum, not replace the teacher's responsibility for delivering PSHE and RSHE. The Department for Education (2021) stresses that schools retain accountability for the content and delivery of their Relationships, Sex and Health Education programmes, meaning any external input should support clearly defined learning objectives.

The National Institute for Health and Care Excellence (NICE) guidance on alcohol interventions in secondary and further education highlights why many teachers welcome external speakers: they are often seen as more engaging and experienced, especially when some staff feel uncertain or uncomfortable delivering sensitive lessons themselves. Yet NICE (2019) also warns that the impact of external speakers can vary significantly. Some visitors may lack the necessary skills to connect meaningfully with young people, reducing the session's effectiveness. This undermines the importance of teachers remaining at the centre of substance education. They know their pupils best, understand the school's ethos and are able to weave teaching into the broader curriculum and whole-school culture. External contributors should be invited only after thorough vetting to ensure their approach aligns with school policies, safeguarding requirements and curriculum aims.

A well-planned collaboration means external visitors enhance rather than disrupt learning, offering specialist knowledge or real-world insights that teachers might not have. This approach safeguards consistency and supports pupils' understanding by embedding lessons within a sequenced, spiral curriculum that builds knowledge and skills over time. Effective substance education depends on strong teacher leadership, with external contributors playing a supportive role. This should be a partnership that enriches learning while keeping the school's vision and pupils' needs firmly in view.

Strategies for Delivering Substance Education Effectively

When teaching about substances, it's essential to create a learning environment where pupils feel psychologically safe, respected and able to express themselves without fear of judgement.

Creating Learner Agreements

One of the most effective ways to do this is by co-creating a learner agreement at the very start of the topic.

Rather than presenting pupils with a fixed set of ground rules, I find it much more powerful to develop this agreement *with* them. It's important that pupils understand that both teacher and pupils have a responsibility to treat each other sensitively. By doing this collaboratively, we help create a shared understanding that everyone in the room has rights and responsibilities, including the teacher.

In the first session, I'll typically introduce the session theme (for example, drugs or alcohol) so pupils are clear about what we'll be discussing. Then I'll bring up the idea of a learner agreement and ask pupils to suggest what would help them feel comfortable and respected in discussions. This can be done as a class brainstorm on the board using sentence starters or prompts like

- What helps you feel safe to share your thoughts?
- How should we treat each other during these lessons?

From there, we build an agreement together. A good one might include

- Be confidential (but understand the limits of confidentiality).
- Only speak if you feel comfortable.

- Respect others' views and feelings.
- Use kind, non-judgemental language.
- Avoid language that others may find offensive or derogatory.
- Remember that if something is shared that suggests a pupil is at risk, it will be reported (safeguarding always comes first).

This agreement is usually displayed on the board or on a dedicated slide throughout the topic. If the conversation ever becomes difficult or a boundary is crossed, I gently remind pupils of the agreement by returning to the slide, not to shame, but to re-centre ourselves. It's a simple but effective way of reinforcing the tone of the space we've created together.

Anonymous Q&A and Classroom Safety

One of the most effective ways to create a safe and inclusive learning environment when teaching about harmful substances is to use anonymous question strategies. These strategies are not just a useful classroom technique, they're also a way of ensuring that every pupil has a voice, not just the confident few. In my experience, anonymous question tools allow pupils to access information in a way that feels safer and more manageable. They remove the fear of judgement, shame or stigma and can open up discussions that might otherwise be left unsaid. Sometimes, during open classroom conversations, it's the same pupils who tend to speak up. While their contributions are valuable, they shouldn't be the only voices we hear. Anonymous Q&A strategies make it possible for the quieter pupils, those who are curious but cautious, to take part and have their questions answered.

I usually hand out Post-it notes at the beginning of the lesson. This is important because if pupils have a question midway through, they can write it down without worrying they'll forget it later. I give them a clear structure: write the question, fold the paper twice and place it in the box. This routine helps normalise the process, and it signals to pupils that their thoughts are valued and treated respectfully. I don't typically answer the questions during the same lesson. Instead, I review them after the lesson and respond to them the following week. This gives me time to check that questions are appropriate to read aloud and, if I need to, do a bit of research myself. When I present the answers, I'll explain the source of my information, often modelling how to use a reliable website or resource. This is a key opportunity to show pupils how to question what they read online and avoid misinformation. If several questions touch on the same theme, I'll use that as a prompt for future planning, either by building it into the next session or weaving it through other lessons. Any question that raises a safeguarding concern is shared immediately with the DSL, along with details of the class and context. We can't always know who wrote the note, but we can take what's shared seriously and act on it appropriately.

Avoiding Scare Tactics and Using Evidence

One of the most important things to get right when teaching about harmful substances is your tone. Young people are very sharp. They can spot sensationalism a mile off, and scare tactics can often backfire. Rather than discouraging risky behaviour, they can breed mistrust or even spark curiosity. As **Notts Alone** puts it,

> Teenagers often know more about drugs than you do, so there's no point in saying, 'Smoking cannabis will kill you.' Pointing out that cannabis can cause mental health problems, especially if you start smoking it in your teens, may be more of a deterrent.

In my experience, it's always best to give pupils the facts in a calm, neutral way. I treat this kind of teaching partially like a science lesson. These are the substances. These are the short- and long-term physical effects and these are the impacts on mental health. By taking this clinical, fact-based approach, I avoid moralising or preaching, which can alienate pupils and shut down meaningful dialogue. Once I've laid out the factual, biological effects, I then shift the focus and invite pupils to explore the wider impact. What could the social, psychological, financial or emotional consequences of substance use look like? This part of the session usually prompts deeper thinking and a lot of insightful discussion. Pupils will often highlight how substance misuse doesn't just harm the individual but can have a ripple effect, hurting families, friends, relationships and opportunities. When they reach these conclusions for themselves, it's far more powerful than anything I could have told them.

Using evidence from trusted sources like NHS Digital, Talk to Frank or YoungMinds is essential. It not only builds your credibility, but it also models to pupils how to seek out reliable, accurate information themselves. It also helps protect you professionally, especially when dealing with sensitive or contested topics. The aim isn't to shock pupils into obedience. We want to equip them with knowledge, skills and critical thinking so they can make informed decisions that are right for them.

Engaging Delivery Techniques

When teaching about substances, the way we deliver the content can make all the difference. For pupils to engage meaningfully with the topic, we need to strike a balance between being informative and making space for active participation and reflection. In my experience, using videos or short case studies can be a powerful way to anchor discussions. These resources bring the topic to life and often act as a mirror for pupils to recognise real-life situations they or their peers might face. If a young person can see the humanity in someone's story, rather than a lecture, they're much more likely to listen, connect and reflect.

Role play is another technique I use regularly. Some pupils find it awkward at first, but with the right structure and safe classroom climate, it becomes an opportunity for them to practise handling peer pressure in a way that's realistic. The beauty of role play is that it gives pupils a chance to try out different responses, hear feedback from their peers and gain the confidence they'll need in real-life situations. I also like to start some lessons with a sorting or categorising activity. It's quick, simple and helps me gauge what pupils already know or think they know. Activities like 'strongest to weakest influence' spark conversation and surface misunderstandings in a non-threatening way. You can do this by getting pupils to rank different influences on a person's decision to use or avoid substances from 'strongest to weakest influence.' For example, they might consider peer pressure, family attitudes, media messaging, personal values or access to substances.

This activity encourages thoughtful discussion and helps pupils realise that influence isn't always obvious or direct. It also gives them space to reflect on what (or who) shapes their own decisions, which can be a powerful step toward developing personal resilience and critical thinking. This type of strategy also works well in pairs or small groups and can build oracy skills too. The key is to keep lessons interactive and relevant. Pupils need to feel that their voice matters and that they're not just being talked at. They need to feel like they are a part of the learning journey.

Use of Retrieval, Oracy and Reading in Delivery

Effective substance education relies not only on what we teach but how we help pupils engage with, remember and reflect on that content. Retrieval practice, oracy and inclusive use of texts and visuals all play an important part in ensuring lessons are not only understood in the moment but remembered long after they leave the classroom.

Retrieval practice is about helping pupils bring prior knowledge to mind so it can be built upon. It's not just a memory exercise; it's an essential learning strategy. That said, not all retrieval activities are created equal. In an Education Endowment Foundation (EEF) blog *Retrieval practice – A common good or just commonplace?* (2021), Professor Rob Coe cautions that if tasks are too simple, they might not stretch pupils' thinking far enough to actually enhance memory or deepen understanding. Based on this, I tend to avoid multiple-choice quizzes during KS4 when teaching about substances. These often offer too much of a prompt and don't truly measure what pupils have remembered.

Instead, I prefer sentence starters like 'Give an example of . . .' or 'List three types of. . . .' These push pupils to think more deeply and actively recall information from previous lessons. I sometimes display key vocabulary on the board and ask pupils to explain it in their own words or link terms together. The aim here is not rote recall but thoughtful engagement.

The EEF blog also suggests that if we want pupils to become confident with higher-order questions, we can adapt our retrieval tasks accordingly by asking them to explain, analyse or evaluate, rather than simply recall. I've found this approach encourages more meaningful conversations and often reveals what pupils really understand, beyond surface-level facts. One activity I've used involves giving pupils a statement like 'Drinking alcohol affects decision-making' and asking them to explain how or why this is the case. It's a small shift, but it opens the door to higher-order thinking and supports meaningful discussion. It also highlights any misconceptions which can then be addressed in the moment. Effective retrieval practice isn't about testing the pupils. It's about strengthening learning, making connections and helping pupils feel confident in what they know.

Promoting Oracy and Discussion

Substance education isn't just about knowing the facts. It's also about being able to talk about them. Oracy plays a central role in helping pupils articulate their values, reflect on peer influence and develop strategies for real-life situations. However, getting everyone involved in discussion takes planning and sensitivity. There are a number of ways pupils are able to participate in the lesson. One strategy I often use is *Think–Pair–Share*. According to Edutopia (2023), this method gives all pupils a chance to think quietly before being asked to speak. After a short pause to reflect, they share their ideas with a partner before opening up to the wider group. This routine helps to 'create equity of voice' and reduces pressure, especially for quieter pupils or those who may feel unsure about speaking in front of the class.

Another useful strategy is 'thinking routines.' Pupils work in small groups to respond to open-ended prompts like 'Why do you think people take risks with substances?' or 'What might influence someone to say no?' These routines are more than just conversation starters. They help me to gather insights into what pupils think and feel. The information they share can be used to adapt future lesson plans, ensuring the curriculum stays relevant and responsive to their needs. Even more importantly, they can be used for whole-school initiatives. Respectful listening should also be heavily promoted by using phrases like 'good listening' and reminding pupils to show respect when someone shares. Over time, this fosters a class culture where everyone feels heard and respected. Sometimes I use a formal debate format, giving pupils the chance to express opposing views while learning how to disagree respectfully. This builds confidence and helps pupils develop critical thinking. These are the skills they'll need when navigating difficult choices in real life.

Using Texts and Visuals Inclusively

When selecting reading materials, images or videos, it's essential that pupils see themselves reflected and that no one feels excluded, judged or stereotyped. Inclusive teaching isn't about ticking boxes; it's about creating a space where every pupil feels like they belong and where a diverse range of experiences and voices are explored with care. Resources should be chosen that represent different backgrounds, identities and experiences. This could mean using case studies with varied family dynamics or videos that feature young people from different ethnic and socio-economic groups. It's about showing that substance use, and the choices surrounding it, affect people in a range of contexts.

Sometimes texts can be used that show how someone's environment, relationships or mental health played a role in their choices. These narratives help pupils develop empathy and understand that there's rarely a single cause behind someone's behaviour. Visuals that are up-to-date and free from scare tactics or stigmatising language are also another important factor. When we read or watch something together, pupils should be given time to pause and respond, either in writing or through discussion. Pupils are encouraged to use mini whiteboards to write down their responses. I'll ask questions such as, 'What do you notice?' or 'How might different people experience this differently?' These moments encourage critical thinking and help pupils to unpack the messages they're receiving.

Most importantly, I'm mindful not to present any one experience as universal. Substance use, addiction and recovery are complex, and our resources should reflect that complexity with care and balance. By doing this, we make space for every pupil to engage in a way that feels respectful, inclusive and real.

Spiral Learning, Curriculum Integration and Cross-Topic Links

One of the most effective ways to embed substance education is through a spiral curriculum, which is a model where key concepts are revisited at increasing levels of complexity and depth over time. Rather than delivering one-off sessions or isolated topics, a spiral approach supports sustained understanding by building on what pupils already know and ensuring they revisit essential content at appropriate developmental stages. An excellent starting point is the PSHE Association's thematic model, which maps out key concepts across Key Stages in a sequenced and age-appropriate way. For example, in Year 7, pupils are introduced to how to manage influences relating to substances such as caffeine, smoking and alcohol during the spring term. This is typically taught as a stand-alone lesson, laying the groundwork with core facts and an understanding of personal responsibility.

By Year 8, in the autumn term, this learning is deepened significantly. Pupils explore a full topic on 'Drugs and Alcohol,' which includes more complex ideas such as drug misuse, peer pressure and habit versus dependency. This unit moves beyond the basics to include learning about medicinal and recreational drugs; the safe use of prescription and over-the-counter medication; and the physical and psychological effects of alcohol, tobacco, nicotine and e-cigarettes. It also encourages pupils to critically reflect on social norms, challenge stigma and consider the broader impacts of substance use on relationships and well-being.

This is a strong example of what spiral learning looks like in practice in PSHE. The Year 7 lesson introduces influences and decisions, and the Year 8 unit revisits this with greater depth and relevance to pupils' lives as they mature. Not only do they consolidate prior learning, but they also gain new strategies for managing increasing levels of risk. In a well-sequenced spiral curriculum, certain concepts, such as managing influence, recognising risks and understanding the law, are revisited again and again. However, each return to the topic should offer pupils something new: an opportunity to apply their knowledge to a different context or to reflect more deeply based on new experiences or growing maturity.

It's also worth noting that in a spiral model, timing matters. Ensuring the right content is delivered at the right point in a pupil's development is essential for it to be meaningful. Some pupils might not yet be exposed to peer pressure or substances in Year 7, but they need the tools and language in advance, not in reaction. A spiral curriculum isn't about repetition for the sake of it. It's about creating a cohesive journey where substance education becomes part of pupils' developing identity, values and critical thinking. When done well, it ensures that vital messages aren't just delivered, they're remembered.

Reinforcing Substance Education Across Subjects

In my teaching of PSHE, substance education rarely sits in isolation from other subjects. With a primary teaching background, I've always approached PSHE through an interdisciplinary lens, drawing from across the curriculum to enrich, embed and bring the learning to life. In fact, I genuinely believe any subject can reinforce the messages and skills we're trying to build around substance use and personal safety. Drama, for example, is a powerful way to explore social pressures and practice managing influences in a safe, creative space. Role play gives pupils the opportunity to step into real-life scenarios, test out responses and receive feedback, not just from me, but from their peers too. It builds empathy, confidence and a deeper understanding of how situations can unfold.

I've also used art and media to explore themes like vaping. In one lesson, pupils created their own advertising campaigns. Some were tasked with encouraging vaping, others with discouraging it. At first glance, this might sound counterintuitive. But there's a reason behind it. The reality is that young people are being targeted by e-cigarette companies every day. From sweet flavours to bright packaging, the tactics are deliberate and effective. By designing their own brand campaigns, pupils come to understand these strategies and how they manipulate appeal and bypass logic. They then begin to think critically about the media they consume. We usually start by analysing a mix of pro- and anti-vaping adverts before splitting into two creative teams. It's playful but purposeful, and the discussion that follows is often just as insightful as the task itself. Careful preparation is essential to making these lessons effective and meaningful. For example, when planning the media analysis and advertising task, it's important to source a range of real-world adverts that reflect both sides of the argument, those promoting vaping and those warning against it. This gives pupils the tools to explore the contrast between persuasive marketing techniques and public health messaging, and it encourages them to engage with the issue from multiple angles. High-quality resources also help avoid presenting a one-sided or overly simplistic view. Whether it's curating appropriate visuals, designing scenario cards or ensuring scientific accuracy, thoughtful preparation enables pupils to build critical thinking skills, make informed choices and connect the content to their everyday lives.

Of course, science, particularly biology and chemistry, offers a natural home for substance education. Understanding how drugs, alcohol and tobacco affect the brain and body gives pupils the factual grounding they need. When we've already laid that scientific foundation, PSHE lessons can focus on social and emotional learning, values and decision-making. Citizenship is another space where substance-related issues can be explored through discussion, rights and responsibilities. Debates can be facilitated around drug policy, age restrictions and the ethics of legalisation. These conversations help pupils develop their own views while practising respectful dialogue and critical thinking.

Even geography has a place. As we develop young people into global citizens, it's vital they understand that laws and norms differ around the world. What's legal in one country may be criminal in another. These insights promote a more nuanced understanding of culture, law and behaviour. The truth is substance education becomes much more meaningful when it's threaded through a pupil's whole school experience. That's the beauty of a well-integrated curriculum. Pupils start to see the links, make connections, and most importantly, understand the 'why' behind the learning. Whether it's debating in citizenship, role-playing in drama or analysing ad campaigns in art, every subject can play its part in building pupils' knowledge, resilience and decision-making skills.

Cross-Topic Connections

The choices pupils make about smoking, drinking, vaping or experimenting with other substances are deeply connected to their health, emotions, relationships, values and goals. That's why substance education works best when it's woven into a bigger picture, rather than treated as a standalone topic.

This book sits alongside nine other themes in the PSHE Toolkit series. While each topic can be taught in isolation, there are strong and natural overlaps that can deepen PSHE learning. Next, I've highlighted some key connections between substance education and the rest of the PSHE Toolkit, along with practical ways to bring those links into your teaching.

Mental Health

Many young people are exposed to substances in the context of stress, anxiety, peer pressure or low self-esteem. There's often a link between how someone feels and how they cope, and for some, harmful substances may appear to offer relief, escape or control.

Throughout the *Harmful Substances* lessons, you can make gentle links back to **mental health strategies** covered elsewhere. For example,

- When discussing why people might turn to substances, acknowledge emotions like loneliness, anxiety or pressure to fit in.
- Reinforce healthy coping strategies: talking to someone, exercise, journaling, breathing techniques or creative outlets.
- Explore how substances might impact mental health long-term, particularly for young people still developing emotionally and neurologically.

This connection helps pupils understand that substance misuse is rarely just about the substance. It's often about what's going on underneath the surface.

Relationships Education

Substance use often intersects with relationships. Whether it's the influence of peers, dynamics in a friendship group, romantic pressure or family environments, young people rarely make choices in isolation.

You can strengthen links with **relationships education** by

- Exploring **consent** in the context of substances. What happens to someone's ability to consent when under the influence of alcohol or drugs?
- Discussing **peer pressure** and how to handle situations where friends or partners encourage risky behaviour.
- Encouraging pupils to think about **boundaries** and respect, both for themselves and others.

The goal isn't to frame every discussion as a warning, but to give pupils the language and confidence to recognise when situations feel uncomfortable and know how to respond.

Media Literacy

There is a huge overlap between harmful substances and **media literacy**. Advertising, films, music and social media all play a role in shaping young people's ideas about smoking, drinking and drug use.

In your substance education lessons, encourage pupils to

- Analyse the messages behind adverts for alcohol or vaping products.
- Think critically about the role of substances in TV, film and music. Are they being romanticised or treated as normal?
- Consider what's missing from those portrayals: the consequences, regrets, health issues or emotional fallout.

You could also make connections to online safety by

- Spotting misinformation or glamorisation of drugs and alcohol on platforms like TikTok, Snapchat or Instagram.
- Discussing the risks of buying substances online or sharing images/videos while under the influence.
- Reinforcing critical thinking: Who's posting this? Why? What don't we see behind the scenes?

Connecting media literacy and online safety helps pupils develop a more realistic understanding of how substances are portrayed online and how those messages can influence behaviour. These lessons empower pupils to make more informed, less reactive decisions in a world full of persuasive messages. Online spaces are increasingly part of how young people encounter harmful substances: through influencers, social media trends, private group chats or even illegal sales.

Sex Education

Sexual activity and substance use can be closely linked, especially as young people grow older and start socialising more independently. Alcohol and drugs can impact **judgement, consent, memory and safety**, which are all key themes covered in sex education.

You can build on this by

- Highlighting how substances affect someone's ability to give or interpret consent.
- Opening space for reflection on how people might behave differently when under the influence and what risks that might introduce.
- Reinforcing respect for personal boundaries and decision-making, no matter the context.

The overlap here isn't always comfortable, but it is essential. The aim is never to scare pupils, but to equip them to recognise risky situations and protect themselves and others.

Physical Health

Of course, the most immediate and visible connection is with **physical health**. Lessons around substances naturally link to topics like the respiratory system, liver function, addiction and long-term well-being.

To strengthen this connection,

- Include discussions on how vaping affects the lungs or how alcohol impacts the brain.
- Reinforce positive habits such as hydration, sleep and exercise as protective factors.
- Emphasise that health isn't just about avoiding harm, but actively building strength, energy and resilience.

Physical health knowledge gives pupils a scientific foundation for understanding why substances can be harmful, even if those effects aren't always obvious straight away.

Financial Education

Substances can come with a real cost . . . literally. Linking with **finance education**, you can explore

- How much someone might spend weekly or monthly on vaping or drinking.
- What else could that money go toward?
- How substances might affect a person's ability to manage money or hold down a job in the future.

While gambling may feel like a separate issue, the **risk-taking mindset** behind it can mirror the thinking behind substance use. Both can be impulsive, emotionally driven and socially influenced. They can also both trigger short-term rewards but lead to long-term consequences. These conversations help pupils see the wider consequences of their choices, including how substance use can affect future plans and financial independence. They also see how addiction can appear in all forms, not just related to drugs and alcohol.

You can draw the connection by

- Discussing the psychology of addiction and how dopamine works in both gambling and substance misuse.
- Exploring peer influence and social media pressures in both areas.
- Reinforcing refusal skills, boundaries and how to get help if things start to feel out of control.

Careers

Substance misuse can directly affect **future opportunities**, and this is where careers education ties in:

- Talk openly about how substance use might impact applications, interviews or performance in jobs and apprenticeships.
- Encourage pupils to reflect on what kind of jobs exist to create better opportunities for people with addictions.
- Highlight success stories and role models from different careers who've made positive choices, especially those who've overcome challenges or spoken out about addiction.

Helping pupils connect today's decisions to tomorrow's possibilities makes the learning feel real and gives them something to aim for.

Personal Safety

The **personal safety** strand is closely aligned with substance education. In fact, many of the risks that come with harmful substances (loss of control, impaired judgement, dangerous settings) are core personal safety concerns.

Ways to link these areas are as follows:

- Discuss scenarios where substance use increases risk, e.g. walking home intoxicated, accepting a drink from someone or feeling unsafe but unable to speak up.
- Reinforce refusal strategies: assertive communication, body language and trusting your gut instincts.
- Address the blurred lines between safety and social pressure, helping pupils practise recognising uncomfortable situations and making exit plans.

This helps pupils place their safety at the centre of decision-making, even when social dynamics make that feel hard.

First Aid

Sometimes substance use leads to real emergencies, either through overdose, allergic reaction, injury or unconsciousness. This is where your **first aid** strand becomes highly relevant.

Build the connection by

- Exploring what signs to look out for if someone has consumed too much alcohol, is unconscious or is struggling to breathe.
- Discussing when and how to call for help and that pupils will never be in trouble for doing the right thing in an emergency.
- Revisiting the recovery position, checking for breathing and knowing what to say when speaking to emergency services.

This gives young people practical tools they can draw on in moments of crisis and could literally save lives.

Linking topics together isn't about cramming everything into one lesson. It's about weaving threads across the year so that learning feels joined up, relevant and grounded in real life. Substance education is part of a much bigger picture. When we connect it to issues like identity, emotions, safety and aspirations, we help young people build the skills, confidence and insight to make informed decisions, not just about substances, but about life.

Long-Term Learning and Cohesion

When we think about long-term learning in PSHE, particularly in substance education, it's not just about what pupils remember, it's about how they grow more confident and capable with each revisit of a concept. A strong, spiralled curriculum doesn't just re-teach the same content. It deepens and stretches pupils' understanding year after year, helping them to apply prior knowledge to new and more complex situations. For example, in Year 8, after covering the topic of drugs and alcohol in the autumn term, pupils go on in the spring term to explore how to manage influences on beliefs and decisions, including themes like group-think and persuasion in relation to discrimination. While I can't recall a single conversation or moment, what stands out is how the pupils begin to act. During role-play activities, they often show strong assertiveness, and this confidence often feels like a direct result of the groundwork laid earlier in the year. They've practised navigating peer pressure before, and now they're not only remembering those lessons, but they're also using them. This kind of visible progression reinforces why it's so important not to rush through topics. When we allow time for reflection, revisit key skills like resistance strategies and encourage pupils to link ideas across terms or even across years, the learning sticks.

Sometimes, lessons take unexpected turns: a spontaneous discussion or an unplanned moment of honesty, and rather than seeing this as a detour, this can be seen as part of the learning journey. The most meaningful teaching often happens in these moments of connection, where pupils see how everything links: from their science lessons on the effects of substances, to debates in citizenship, to real-life pressures outside the school gates. This is the power of cohesion. It's what makes PSHE more than a series of lessons. It makes it a series of lessons as part of a young person's life education.

Teaching Substance Education in International and Traditional Contexts

Substance education can feel like one of the most culturally sensitive topics to teach, especially in international schools or communities with strong religious or traditional values. Attitudes toward alcohol, smoking, drugs and even mental health can differ widely depending on local laws, belief systems and cultural norms. This is the reason why this curriculum has been designed to offer structure and guidance while also allowing room for flexibility and cultural relevance. In some schools, alcohol may be illegal or entirely absent from community life. In others, young people might be exposed to substances far earlier, through social events, older siblings or online influencers. Rather than assume one cultural 'norm,' this book encourages teachers to create safe, respectful learning spaces where the focus is always on well-being, informed choices and critical thinking.

The legal status of substances like cannabis, energy drinks, tobacco or even prescribed medication varies around the world. However, the risks associated with misuse remain the same and so does the need for pupils to develop key life skills, such as recognising influence, thinking critically about risk and understanding the effects substances can have on both body and mind. Where legal and social rules differ, the content of a lesson can be adapted but the intention stays the same: to help young people make safe, respectful and informed decisions that support their health and personal values.

If you're working in a school where certain substances are never mentioned at home or are considered taboo, you may choose to adapt the vocabulary or use broader terms. For example, you might focus on 'harmful influences' or 'pressure to take risks' rather than naming specific drugs. You might also replace examples with local or culturally relevant alternatives, especially if talking about alcohol or drug misuse feels too direct. There's no one-size-fits-all script for these conversations, but the structure and objectives of each lesson in this book can be easily adapted to suit different school environments. Balancing cultural respect with student safeguarding is a key part of teaching substance education in global and traditional settings. There may be pupils who come from homes where substance use is heavily stigmatised or simply not talked about. Others may have been exposed to substances early in life but are unsure where to go for support.

Creating a non-judgemental, inclusive space is vital. You don't need to challenge cultural values, but you do need to ensure that pupils are safe, informed and able to seek help if they need it. This is especially true if they're being exposed to harm in silence. If you're concerned that a student may be at risk, follow your school's safeguarding policy. In any school or setting, student welfare must always come first. Substance education isn't just about drugs or alcohol. It is also about developing a broader understanding of personal responsibility, media literacy, health and respect. These are universal values. Whether you're teaching in London, Lagos, Dubai or Singapore, helping pupils explore these issues builds their capacity to make thoughtful choices, respect different perspectives and navigate real-world pressures.

Young people in international schools are often negotiating multiple cultural identities. They may hear one message at school, another at home and yet another from TikTok. Giving them a space to explore, question and reflect is not only powerful, but it's also protective.

Challenges and Professional Development for Staff

One of the most common concerns teachers face when delivering substance education is the fear of getting something wrong like saying the wrong thing or giving out incorrect information. This fear can make teachers feel unsure about their ability to lead lessons on what can be a high-stakes, emotionally loaded topic. Personally, I've always felt quite comfortable teaching this area, but I remember early on worrying whether I had enough subject knowledge to deliver the facts accurately. What helped was building my confidence over time, through continuing professional development (CPD), through learning from external experts and simply through experience and repetition in the classroom.

This topic becomes even more challenging if a teacher has personal experience with drug or alcohol misuse, either their own or through close family or friends. In these cases, the topic can feel particularly triggering. It's vital that teachers give themselves permission to teach in a way that feels manageable and safe for them. This might mean taking extra care with lesson content, seeking support from colleagues or asking for alternative arrangements when needed. Pupils may also ask personal questions, especially if they feel curious or connected to the topic. It's important to maintain boundaries. You should always let pupils know that your role is to guide them through the facts and help them explore the topic thoughtfully, not to share your personal history. Keeping the pupil–adult dynamic clear and respectful is key.

Disclosures are another important challenge. If a pupil shares something concerning, it's crucial that teachers know their school's safeguarding policy inside and out and that they follow it consistently. Some pupils may also test boundaries with inappropriate comments or poor behaviour, which can undermine the seriousness of the topic. This is where a strong learner agreement becomes essential. It will give you something to return to when those moments arise, reminding everyone of the shared expectations. Above all, remember that every pupil brings their own lived experience. For some, this may include trauma, cultural beliefs or social norms around substances that differ from what's typically discussed in school. Teaching this topic requires a high level of cultural and social sensitivity and a willingness to approach every conversation with care and compassion.

CPD and Support for Confidence Building

Building confidence to teach about drugs, alcohol and other harmful substances doesn't happen overnight. For many teachers, especially those without a specialist background in health or PSHE, the idea of covering such a complex and sensitive topic can feel daunting. This is where high-quality CPD and ongoing support play a vital role. As mentioned previously, what helped me most was attending regular CPD sessions and hearing from external experts. These were people who not only had deep subject knowledge but also practical strategies for engaging pupils and managing sensitive discussions. Sometimes you just need to hear how someone else phrases something or frames a difficult idea in a way that makes sense.

Continuing professional development can cover a range of things, from understanding the latest research on substance use among young people to developing strategies for handling disclosures and maintaining appropriate boundaries. It can also help you build your own language and confidence for talking about substances in a clear and non-judgemental way. Another key benefit of professional development is that it can help you feel less isolated. Talking to other teachers about what's working, and what isn't, reminds you that everyone is figuring this out together. Sharing challenges and successes makes a real difference, especially in a topic where moral judgement or fear of saying the wrong thing can get in the way of progress.

Sometimes, confidence also grows with practice. The more I taught these lessons, the more I developed a rhythm that worked for me, using real-life case studies, interactive activities and open discussions. Over time, I also learned to anticipate the kinds of questions pupils might ask and how to respond without panic, even when they caught me off-guard. What I've also learned is that you don't need to know everything. It's okay to say, 'Let's research it now together and find out,' or to bring in materials from trusted sources to support what you're teaching. CPD isn't about becoming an expert overnight. It is about feeling equipped to hold the space and facilitate learning in a safe and supportive way.

Reflection and Peer Learning

One of the most powerful ways to build staff confidence and competence is through peer learning. Reflecting together after a lesson, sharing what went well and what felt difficult, creates a collaborative and supportive environment. I've learned so much just by listening to a colleague talk through how they handled a challenging question or adapted a lesson on the spot. Structured reflection, whether it's in staff meetings, twilight CPD or peer observations helps normalise the idea that PSHE teaching is a professional skill that needs development like any other. It shouldn't be something we're expected to just 'get on with.'

When teachers reflect together, we also start to spot patterns. These may include what's resonating with pupils, what misconceptions they hold or where the curriculum might need tweaking. This collective insight is invaluable for long-term planning and curriculum improvement. Most importantly, peer learning reminds us that we're not alone. Substance education can be tough, but with the right conversations and consistent support, we can all become more confident, capable and impactful in the classroom.

Teacher FAQs/Tricky Moments

Even with a strong plan, peer learning and inclusive strategies in place, some moments in PSHE lessons can feel uncertain or uncomfortable. It's completely normal to face tricky questions or situations when teaching about harmful substances. The important thing is to stay calm, honest and professional and to remember that you're not expected to have all the answers on the spot. Next are a few common scenarios and ideas on how to handle them.

Q: What if a Student Asks if I've Used Drugs?

It's not uncommon for pupils to test boundaries or try to make the topic more personal. They might be curious or simply trying to provoke a reaction. Whatever the motive, you don't need to share personal information.

A simple response could be

> 'This lesson isn't about my choices, it's about helping you make safe, informed decisions for yourself.'

Keep it neutral, kind and firm. You can also use it as an opportunity to reinforce the learning objective:

> 'I'm here to give you the facts and help you think through what's best for your health and future.'

This keeps the focus on them, where it belongs, without making it a personal disclosure.

Q: What if I Disagree With the Curriculum?

It's perfectly okay to have personal opinions that differ from parts of the curriculum. However, when teaching PSHE, it's important to present the content in a balanced, professional way that reflects statutory guidance and the school's agreed framework.

If something doesn't sit right with you, try to focus on facilitating discussion rather than pushing a particular viewpoint. For example, try saying,

> 'Different people and cultures have different beliefs about this. Let's look at the facts and talk about the impact substances can have, so you can make your own informed decisions.'

You can also speak to your PSHE lead or line manager outside the classroom if you feel strongly about particular content. There might be flexibility in how things are delivered, as long as the core messages are still covered.

Q: What if I Suspect a Parent Is Supplying Substances?

This is a safeguarding concern and must be taken seriously. You don't need to investigate, and you definitely should not confront anyone yourself. Your responsibility is to report it to the appropriate safeguarding lead in your school as soon as possible.

Stick to the facts: what you've seen, heard or noticed. Even if you're unsure, it's always safer to raise a concern and let trained staff take it forward. The DSL will know the right steps to take, and your role is to pass the information on promptly and confidentially.

Q: What if a Student Tells Me They've Used Substances?

If a student discloses that they've used drugs, alcohol or another harmful substance, stay calm and listen without judgement. Thank them for being honest and avoid reacting in a way that could make them feel ashamed or shut down.

It's important not to make promises you can't keep. You might say something like,

> 'I'm really glad you told me. I want to make sure you're safe, so I may need to speak to someone who can support you properly.'

Follow your school's safeguarding procedures and refer the concern to the DSL. Don't try to handle it alone. Even if the student asks you not to tell anyone, explain gently that you have a duty to keep them safe.

Q: What if Pupils Laugh or Joke About Substance Misuse?

It's not unusual for pupils to react to difficult topics with humour, discomfort or bravado. Sometimes it's a defence mechanism; other times it's an attempt to test the boundaries. Either way, it's worth addressing calmly and without embarrassment.

You might say,

> 'I understand some people might feel awkward or unsure how to react, but this is a serious topic, and I expect everyone to show respect so we can learn safely.'

This reinforces classroom expectations and protects the tone of the lesson without shutting pupils down. You can always pause and reset the atmosphere or shift to a quieter activity if needed.

What Pupils Told Me About Drug Culture

When I asked a group of Year 10 pupils to share what they knew about how young people experience drug and vape culture today, their responses were direct, insightful and, honestly, pretty eye-opening. They spoke first about vaping. They told me that many vape products are clearly marketed to attract young people, with bright colours, playful packaging and sweet, fruit-flavoured options like strawberry or bubblegum. They shared slang terms I hadn't come across before, like *dolo* (means 'vaping'), and explained that it's incredibly easy for pupils in Year 9 or 10 to access vapes. For those under 13, they admitted it's slightly harder, but still not impossible. Most said that disposable vapes are usually bought from local corner shops or sometimes through peers. Some even mentioned that despite being banned, disposable vapes are still being sold 'under the counter' or via social media. Others admitted that young people often ask older siblings or adults to buy them instead.

When I asked why someone their age might turn to drugs or substances, two reasons stood out again and again**: to forget about life** and **to fit in**. Peer pressure was a consistent theme, whether to look cool, feel included or keep up a certain image. They also reflected on dopamine and the role of social media in all of this. A few of them voiced a worry that platforms like TikTok and Instagram might be 'more addictive than drugs' for some young people, with constant dopamine hits driving the need for validation and escape.

These student voices remind me why we need to centre their lived experiences when we talk about prevention, education and support. They're already thinking critically. We just need to give them the space and trust to be heard.

Final Thoughts

Teaching this topic is about so much more than just delivering facts – it's about being open, sensitive, and creating the kind of environment where pupils feel safe to talk, question and reflect. Yes, there can be challenges, and it's totally normal to feel unsure or worried you'll say the wrong thing. But with a strong curriculum, some creativity and a good learner agreement in place, it's possible to teach this topic in a way that's engaging, respectful and meaningful. You don't need to have all the answers. Just be willing to keep learning, lean on support where you need it and remember that what you're doing really matters.

These lessons won't always be easy, but they will often be the ones pupils remember. You're helping them make sense of the world around them, giving them language for difficult experiences and showing them that support exists. That's powerful. Trust that your care, preparation and willingness to listen make more of an impact than you might realise. Even if you only shift one perspective or start one important conversation, that's enough. Keep showing up, stay human, and remember: education like this doesn't just teach, it empowers.

3 KS3: Lesson Plans

KS3 Lesson 1

<table>
<tr><td>Lesson Title</td><td>Introduction to Harmful Substances</td><td>Key Stage</td><td>3</td></tr>
<tr><td></td><td></td><td>Lesson Length</td><td>50 minutes</td></tr>
<tr><td colspan="4">Lesson Objectives</td></tr>
<tr><td colspan="4">• Define harmful substances and classify common examples into different categories.
• Explain how certain legal substances can still pose health risks.
• Evaluate common misconceptions about harmful substances.
• Describe the basic effects of harmful substances on the body and brain.</td></tr>
<tr><td>Resources Needed</td><td>• Substance sorting worksheet
• Pens and paper
• Post-it notes</td><td>Key Vocabulary</td><td>Harmful substances, legal, illegal, medicinal, recreational, misuse, risk, personal responsibility</td></tr>
<tr><td>Create a Learning Agreement</td><td colspan="3">Begin the lesson by establishing a positive and respectful classroom environment through the creation of a learner agreement. This sets clear expectations for behaviour, participation and respect, helping all pupils feel safe and engaged.

Briefly explain to pupils that the learner agreement is a set of shared rules everyone agrees to follow during the lesson (and ideally, throughout the series). Emphasise that this helps create a respectful space where everyone can learn and express their views safely.

Invite pupils to contribute their ideas about what makes a good learning environment. Prompt with questions like
• What behaviours help us learn best?
• How can we respect each other's opinions?
• What should we do if someone is disruptive?

As pupils suggest behaviours, write these on the board or a visible flipchart. Typical points might include
• Listen when others are speaking.
• Respect different opinions.
• Stay on task and participate.
• Use appropriate language.</td></tr>
</table>

DOI: 10.4324/9781003608998-3

	Read through the list together, clarify any points if needed and ask pupils if they agree. Make adjustments based on consensus to ensure ownership. Write the final learner agreement clearly on a board or handout. Explain that you will refer back to it throughout lessons to maintain a positive learning environment. Have pupils sign a copy of the agreement as a symbolic commitment to the classroom rules (optional). This activity should take approximately 5–7 minutes and sets a respectful tone for the rest of the lessons. The completed learner agreement should be reviewed at the beginning of every lesson.
Starter Activity **(10 minutes)**	Tell pupils you're going to read some statements about substances. • One side of the room = **Agree**, other side = **Disagree**. • Pupils must move physically to the side they most agree with or stand in the middle, if unsure. Introduce the words 'harmful,' 'legal' and 'illegal' to help pupils engage with the Agree/Disagree statements. This will prime their understanding before they discuss. **Harmful**: Something that can cause damage, pain or problems to your body or mind. **Legal**: Something that is allowed by law. **Illegal**: Something that is against the law and not allowed. **Read these statements or choose your own**: • Energy drinks are harmless because you can buy them in shops. • All drugs are illegal. • Vaping is safer than smoking cigarettes. • Some substances can be harmful *even if* they're legal. • You can't become addicted to caffeine. After each statement, ask 1–2 pupils on each side to briefly explain their choice. You could ask • Why do you think that? • Has anyone changed their mind after hearing others speak? **Suggested Explanations** **• Energy drinks are harmless because you can buy them in shops.** False. Just because something is sold legally doesn't mean it's always safe. Energy drinks are high in caffeine and sugar, which can affect sleep, concentration, heart rate and mood, especially for young people.

	• **All drugs are illegal.** Not true. Some drugs, like paracetamol or antibiotics, are legal and used to treat illness. Others, like cannabis (in the United Kingdom), are illegal. It depends on the drug and how it's used. • **Vaping is safer than smoking cigarettes.** Partially true, but not risk-free. Vaping may contain fewer harmful chemicals than cigarettes, but it still affects the lungs and contains addictive nicotine. The long-term health effects are still being studied. • **Some substances can be harmful *even if* they're legal.** True. Legal substances like alcohol, energy drinks and prescription medicines can still harm your health if overused or misused. • **You can't become addicted to caffeine.** False. Caffeine is a stimulant, and some people can become dependent on it. Too much caffeine can lead to headaches, sleep problems and other health issues. **Display or read this explanation about harmful substances aloud and invite pupils to ask clarifying questions.** You could say the following: Harmful substances are things that people put into their bodies, like drugs, medicines, alcohol, certain foods or energy drinks that can cause damage or health problems if used in the wrong way or in large amounts. Some harmful substances are illegal, some are legal but can still be dangerous and others are medicines that help us when used correctly. Understanding these substances helps us make safer choices.
Main Activity (30 minutes)	**Substance Sorting Activity** Give each pair or small group a 'substance sorting worksheet' (**KS3 Lesson 1 Resource 1**). Ask them to sort them into categories you provide (or that they create), such as • Legal versus illegal. • Medicinal versus recreational. • Harmful, if misused versus less harmful (they should discuss as they go). Groups share their categories and explain choices. Teacher leads a discussion to clarify and introduce key vocabulary. Circulate the room, prompting the pupils with questions like • Why did you place this one here? • Can something be both legal and harmful? End with a review of answers and discussion.

	Categories for Sorting Activity • **Alcohol** – Legal (18+)/Recreational/Harmful, if misused • **Paracetamol** – Legal/Medicinal/Harmful, if misused • **Vaping** – Legal (18+)/Recreational/Harmful, if misused • **Energy drinks** – Legal (some shops have a 16+ policy)/Recreational/Harmful, if misused • **Cannabis** – Illegal and legal, in rare cases (18+)/Recreational and medicinal/Harmful, if misused • **Caffeine** – Legal/Recreational/Harmful, if misused • **Antibiotics** – Legal/Medicinal (prescribed by doctor only)/Harmful, if misused • **Social media** – Legal/Recreational/Harmful, if misused (mentally/emotionally) **Extension Task** After the sorting task, ask pupils to work in pairs or small groups to read and discuss the following short scenario: Jamal takes energy drinks before school and again at lunchtime to stay alert. He says it helps him concentrate and feel more awake, but he's been having headaches and trouble sleeping. You could ask • Do you think energy drinks are harmful in this case? Why or why not? • What advice would you give Jamal? • What's the difference between something being *legal* and being *safe*? This discussion helps pupils apply the concepts of harm, legality and personal choice to a relatable real-life situation. Encourage pupils to refer to key vocabulary (e.g. harmful, legal, misuse, personal responsibility) in their responses.
Plenary (10 minutes)	Ask pupils to share one new thing they learned or found surprising from today's lesson. Highlight that harmful substances aren't just illegal drugs but also legal substances that can be misused. Also, reinforce the idea that understanding different categories helps us make safer choices. Display or ask this question for pupils to think about quietly or discuss briefly with a partner: 'Why do you think it's important to know about harmful substances at your age?' Pupils write a short sentence or two as an exit slip: • One thing I learned today is . . . • One question I still have is . . . Alternatively, a quick verbal round where a few volunteers share their sentence aloud.

<table>
<tr>
<td>Assessment Ideas</td>
<td colspan="3">Starter Activity
Use pupil responses during the first activity to assess their baseline understanding and attitudes toward substance use. Listen for clarity, confidence and any signs of uncertainty or misconception. This will help you tailor your input and support during the rest of the lesson.
Main Activity
As pupils work on sorting activities or group tasks, observe how confidently they identify and categorise substances, explain their reasoning and challenge each other's ideas. Pay attention to how they apply knowledge of health impacts, legality and social consequences. Use questioning to encourage critical thinking and note any pupils who may need additional guidance or reinforcement in future lessons.
Plenary
Collect pupils' Post-it notes or written responses from the exit task to gauge the following:
• What key messages they've taken away.
• What questions or uncertainties remain.
• How confident they feel in their understanding.
Look for patterns in responses that highlight misconceptions, emotional reactions or emerging themes worth revisiting. Where appropriate, use these insights to shape the next lesson or provide follow-up clarification.</td>
</tr>
<tr>
<td rowspan="2">Signposting and Support</td>
<td rowspan="2"><u>Website Support</u>
Childline: Free, confidential support for young people.
www.childline.org.uk
Phone: 0800 1111
Talk to Frank: Specialist advice on drugs and alcohol.
www.talktofrank.com
Phone: 0300 123 6600</td>
<td>Cross-Topic Links</td>
<td>Science, media literacy, mental health</td>
</tr>
<tr>
<td>Teaching Tips and Confidence Boosters</td>
<td>Don't worry about having all the answers. If you're unsure, tell pupils you'll find out or encourage them to do safe research (e.g. Talk to Frank, NHS).
Keep the focus on decision-making and safety, not just facts.
Encourage open, respectful discussion. Pupils may have heard different things at home or online.
Use neutral language like 'some people believe . . .' to avoid making pupils feel judged or defensive.</td>
</tr>
</table>

It is good practice to use this example of a reflection prompt after each lesson to help you quickly write down any thoughts after teaching. It's optional but can be helpful for refining future lessons. Use it to note what went well, any challenges, pupil responses or questions and ideas for improvement.

Teacher Reflection

Use this space to write down what went well and what you might change next time.

What parts of the lesson engaged pupils most?

Were there any misconceptions that came up? What might I adapt if I teach this again?

Pupil feedback or notable questions:

KS3 Lesson 2

<table>
<tr><td rowspan="2">Lesson Title:</td><td rowspan="2">Medicinal vs. Recreational Drugs</td><td>Key Stage</td><td>3</td></tr>
<tr><td>Lesson Length:</td><td>50 minutes</td></tr>
<tr><td colspan="4">Lesson Objectives</td></tr>
<tr><td colspan="4">• Explain the difference between medicinal and recreational drugs.
• Identify examples of both types of drugs.
• Understand that some drugs can be used in both ways.
• Recognise potential risks linked to misuse of medicinal and recreational drugs.
• Discuss why medicines should only be taken as prescribed.</td></tr>
<tr><td>Resources Needed</td><td>• Printed statements for the starter activity
• Substance sorting worksheet
• Pens and paper
• Post-it notes</td><td>Key Vocabulary</td><td>Harmful substances, legal, illegal, medicinal, recreational, misuse, risk</td></tr>
<tr><td>Starter Activity (10 minutes)</td><td colspan="3">Review the learner agreement as a class.
Ask this question aloud to the whole class:
'Is medicine the same as a drug? Why do you think that?'
Ask pupils to discuss in pairs or small groups for 2–3 minutes.
Provide guiding prompts on the board or aloud to help them think deeper:
• Can medicines ever be dangerous?
• Are all drugs illegal?
• Is paracetamol a drug? What about alcohol?
Invite a few volunteers to share their group's thinking. Highlight differences, common misconceptions and correct terminology.
You don't need to correct every idea right away. This discussion will naturally lead into defining medicinal versus recreational drugs in the main activity.</td></tr>
<tr><td>Main Activity (30 minutes)</td><td colspan="3">Substance Sorting Activity
Write this list of substances on the board or on a large sheet of paper.
The different categories have been provided here:
• Paracetamol – Medicinal.
• Cannabis – Both (used recreationally and in some medical cases).
• Alcohol – Recreational.
• Antibiotics – Medicinal.
• Cough syrup – Medicinal.
• Cocaine – Recreational (illegal).
• Vaping – Recreational (with addiction risk).</td></tr>
</table>

	• **Diazepam (prescription sedative)** – Medicinal. • **Social media** – Neither, but can be cause addiction (link to dopamine use). Ask pupils to work in pairs or small groups. Their task is to sort each substance (**KS3 Lesson 2 Resource 1**) into one of three categories: • Medicinal. • Recreational. • Both. **Extension Task** Ask pupils to explain their reasoning or note any risks connected to the misuse of each substance. Go through each item as a class. Discuss where it fits and why. Use this time to introduce accurate definitions and correct any misunderstandings. **Key Definitions**: • **Medicinal drug**: A drug used to treat illness or pain, usually prescribed by a doctor or bought from a pharmacy. *Examples: antibiotics, paracetamol* • **Recreational drug**: A drug taken for enjoyment or to change how someone feels. This includes both legal substances (like alcohol) and illegal ones (like cocaine).
Plenary (10 minutes)	You now could say something like Now that we've learned the difference between medicinal and recreational drugs, let's take a moment to think about what this means. I'm going to ask you two questions to reflect on. You can discuss these with a partner or write down your thoughts if you prefer. Ask the following questions to help pupils reflect on the activity they have just completed. • Can a drug be both helpful and harmful? • What makes a drug dangerous? Give pupils 2–3 minutes to discuss these questions in pairs or small groups, or to write down their answers. Invite volunteers to share their thoughts with the class to encourage a brief whole-group discussion. If not already mentioned, remind them that some medicines can help us but also cause harm if misused. It's important to understand both sides. Provide a sentence starter to guide their response, for example, • One thing I learned today about drugs is . . . • A drug can be helpful or harmful because . . .

<table>
<tr><td></td><td colspan="3">Allow 3–5 minutes for pupils to write their answers individually.

Collect what they have written to informally assess understanding and identify any misconceptions to address in future lessons.</td></tr>
<tr><td>Assessment Ideas</td><td colspan="3">Main Activity
While pupils do the sorting task or group discussion, make a note of who can correctly classify substances and who might have misconceptions.

Informal questions like 'Why did you put cannabis in both categories?' help check understanding.

After group sorting, pupils can use peer feedback to explain their choices to another group or pair and receive feedback.

Plenary
Use the responses to give a quick snapshot of individual understanding.</td></tr>
<tr><td rowspan="2">Signposting and Support</td><td rowspan="2"><u>Website Support</u>
NHS Medicines
www.nhs.uk/medicines/

Talk to Frank: Specialist advice on drugs and alcohol.

www.talktofrank.com

Phone: 0300 123 6600

Childline: Free, confidential support for young people.

www.childline.org.uk

Phone: 0800 1111

<u>School Support</u>
Encourage pupils to speak to their school nurse, counsellor or trusted adult if they have questions or concerns about drugs or medicines.</td><td>Cross-Topic Links</td><td>Science (biology), media literacy, citizenship</td></tr>
<tr><td>Teacher Confidence Tips</td><td>Stick to the learning goals. The aim is to help pupils understand that drugs can have different uses, not to list every drug or explain detailed biology.

Encourage discussion. There may be no single 'right' category. Let pupils respectfully debate and explore ideas.

Focus on use and context. Remind pupils that how a substance is used (and why) often determines whether it's helpful or harmful.</td></tr>
</table>

KS3 Lesson 3

<table>
<tr><td rowspan="2">Lesson Title</td><td rowspan="2">Over-Consumption of Energy Drinks</td><td>Key Stage</td><td>3</td></tr>
<tr><td>Lesson Length</td><td>50 minutes</td></tr>
<tr><td colspan="4">Lesson Objectives</td></tr>
<tr><td colspan="4">• Describe what energy drinks are and identify common ingredients (e.g. caffeine, sugar, additives).
• Explain the potential short- and long-term health effects of consuming too many energy drinks.
• Explore why young people might be drawn to energy drinks, including advertising and peer influence.
• Evaluate healthier, more sustainable alternatives for boosting energy and concentration.</td></tr>
<tr><td>Resources Needed</td><td>• Access to YouTube
• A4 or poster paper
• Colouring pens
• Pencils or markers
• Whiteboard and pens</td><td>Key Vocabulary</td><td>Energy drink, caffeine, stimulant, over-consumption, additive, sugar crash, hydration, marketing, health risk</td></tr>
<tr><td>Starter Activity (10 minutes)</td><td colspan="3">Review the learner agreement as a class.

Ask this question aloud:
'What do you already know about energy drinks?'

Encourage pupils to offer any ideas or facts they have. Write pupil responses on the board under the heading 'What we know.' Group similar answers together to keep it organised.

Ask this question next:
'What do you think happens in your body after drinking an energy drink?'

Again, note their responses on the board under 'What happens in the body.'

Prompt pupils to explain or give examples, if needed, and acknowledge all contributions to keep them engaged. Do not correct or evaluate answers at this stage. Save clarifications and myth-busting for later in the lesson.

Keep the recorded answers to use for the plenary.</td></tr>
</table>

<table>
<tr><td>Main Activity (30 minutes)</td><td>Part 1: Watch the video
Introduce the video by saying,
'We're going to watch a short video that explains what energy drinks are, what's inside them and how they can affect your body.'
Play this video for the class:
The Truth About Energy Drinks
https://www.youtube.com/watch?v=l8i9-LiqIy4&t=13s
After watching, ask a few simple questions to check understanding, such as
• What ingredients did you hear about?
• What effects can energy drinks have on the body?
Part 2: Create a warning advert
Explain the task clearly:
'Now, working alone or with a partner, you will design a warning advert or poster to help other young people understand the risks of energy drinks.'
Show or provide key points to include in their advert, based on the video:
• A catchy headline or slogan (for example, 'Think before you drink!').
• Important facts or risks, such as high caffeine or sugar levels and possible health effects.
• Suggestions for healthier choices like water, fruit juice or getting enough sleep.
Provide materials like paper, pens, markers or digital tools if available for creating the adverts. Walk around to support pupils, encourage ideas and ask questions to help them think more deeply.
If time allows, invite some pupils to share their adverts with the class.</td></tr>
</table>

Plenary (10 minutes)	**Revisit the brainstorm from the start of the lesson.** 'Let's look back at our ideas from the beginning of the lesson. Do we still agree with everything here?' 'Would you change or add anything based on what you've learned today?' Encourage pupils to correct any misconceptions or add new information. You might underline ideas that were confirmed, and circle those that were proven incorrect. **Ask these reflection questions out loud (choose one or two):** • What's one thing you learned today that surprised you? • Would you now think twice before having an energy drink? Why or why not? • What's one message from today you'd pass on to a friend? Pupils write one sentence on a Post-it or scrap paper finishing: • One thing I learned today is . . . • One thing I'll remember is . . . They can stick this on the board or hand it in as they leave.
Assessment Ideas	**Starter Activity** Teacher observation during class brainstorm. Note common misconceptions or gaps in knowledge. **Main Activity** Use the verbal responses to video questions. Check for understanding of key points (e.g. What ingredients are in energy drinks? Why might they be harmful?). Support and check pupil adverts. Look for inclusion of key facts, appropriate warnings and clarity of message. If time allows, pairs can swap posters and give one piece of positive feedback and one suggestion for improvement. **Plenary** **Peer feedback (if time allows):** Pairs swap posters and give one piece of positive feedback and one suggestion for improvement.

<table>
<tr>
<td rowspan="2">Signposting and Support</td>
<td rowspan="2"><u>Website Support</u>
Childline: Free, confidential support for young people.
www.childline.org.uk
Phone: 0800 1111
NHS Better Health:
www.nhs.uk/better-health/
YoungMinds: Mental health and well-being resources for young people. Relevant for links between energy drinks, mood swings and anxiety.
www.youngminds.org.uk
Food Standards Agency (FSA): Offers facts on ingredients and health concerns around food and drinks, including caffeine guidelines.
www.food.gov.uk</td>
<td>Cross-Topic Links</td>
<td>Science, maths, media studies, English, citizenship, mental health</td>
</tr>
<tr>
<td>Teacher Confidence Tips</td>
<td>Focus on messages, not memorising facts.
The takeaway should be as follows: too much of something (even legal) can still have risks. If pupils understand that, the lesson is a success.
Let pupils speak.
Use group or class discussion to your advantage. Pupils often have strong opinions about energy drinks. Allow them to explore safely, and guide them back to the facts when needed.
Use questions to guide, not correct.
If a pupil shares a misconception (e.g. 'energy drinks are good for sports'), gently challenge it.</td>
</tr>
</table>

KS3 Lesson 4

<table>
<tr><td rowspan="2">Lesson Title</td><td rowspan="2">The Risks of Vaping and E-Cigarettes</td><td>Key Stage</td><td>3</td></tr>
<tr><td>Lesson Length</td><td>50 minutes</td></tr>
<tr><td colspan="4">Lesson Objectives</td></tr>
<tr><td colspan="4">• Understand the main health risks of vaping.
• Learn how vaping works and what chemicals are involved.
• Recognise why vaping can be addictive, especially for young people.
• Challenge common myths about vaping being safe.</td></tr>
<tr><td>Resources Needed</td><td>• Access to YouTube
• Whiteboard or flip chart
• Pens and paper or exercise books</td><td>Key Vocabulary</td><td>Vaping, nicotine, addiction, chemicals, lung damage, immune system, heart attack, cancer, COPD (chronic obstructive pulmonary disease), pneumothorax</td></tr>
<tr><td>Starter Activity (10 minutes)</td><td colspan="3">Review the learner agreement as a class.

Explain that pupils will complete a short true or false quiz about vaping to see what they already know.

1. Ask pupils to stand or raise their hands to vote for each answer (e.g. True = hands up, False = hands down).
2. After each question, reveal the correct answer and give a brief explanation (provided in this lesson plan).
3. Encourage pupils to share what they think or have heard before giving your explanation.

Here are some questions and explanations you could use:

• Vaping is just water vapour, so it's harmless.
False: Vapes contain chemicals like nicotine, flavourings and fine particles that can harm the lungs.

• Some vapes have more nicotine than a whole pack of cigarettes.
True: Especially with disposable vapes, some contain very high nicotine levels.

• You have to be 18 to buy a vape legally in the United Kingdom.
True: Like tobacco, vapes are illegal to sell to anyone under 18.

• Vaping helps you breathe better than smoking.
False: Vaping still affects lung health and breathing, especially for young people.

• Most teenagers don't vape.
True: While it may seem common, the majority of teens don't vape.</td></tr>
</table>

Main Activity (30 minutes)	Show the whole class the video *The Weird Thing about Vaping You Didn't Know* (https://www.youtube.com/watch?v=as6_ITES1aY). Ask pupils to watch carefully and focus on the information shared. Divide the class into small groups of 3–4 pupils. Give each group these five discussion questions: • What are some common myths about vaping mentioned in the video? • How does vaping affect the lungs and heart, according to the video? • Why is nicotine addictive, and how does vaping keep people hooked? • What serious health problems did the video describe in people who vaped? • After watching, do you think vaping is safer than smoking? Why or why not? Groups talk about each question together and write down key points on paper or whiteboards. After 15–20 minutes, bring the class back together. Ask each group to share their answers to one or two questions. Lead a short class discussion to help deepen everyone's understanding. Finish the activity by summarising the main ideas, focusing on the health risks of vaping and the importance of making informed choices.
Plenary (10 minutes)	Give each pupil a small piece of paper or ask them to write this down: • One new fact they learned about vaping today. • One question they still have or something they want to learn more about. Invite a few pupils to share their answers aloud. Collect their responses to review their understanding and plan any follow-up.
Assessment Ideas	**Starter Activity** Use the quiz at the start to gauge prior knowledge and misconceptions about vaping. **Main Activity** Observe and note pupils' contributions during the video discussion and brainstorm. Look for understanding of key concepts and ability to explain risks. Observe pupils' participation and quality of contributions during the discussion to assess comprehension and critical thinking. **Plenary** Review pupils' written reflections on one new fact learned and any remaining questions. This shows individual understanding and engagement. Ask targeted questions during plenary or the lesson wrap-up to check understanding and correct any misconceptions.

Signposting and Support	**Website Support** **NHS Smokefree**: Tips on quitting smoking and vaping safely. www.nhs.uk/smokefree **Talk to Frank**: Information on drugs including vaping and how to get help. www.talktofrank.com Phone: 0300 123 6600 **YoungMinds**: Support for mental health, which can be linked to addiction and stress. www.youngminds.org.uk **We Are With You**: Advice for substance use, including vaping. www.wearewithyou.org.uk	**Cross-Topic Links**	Science (biology), citizenship, English, mental health
		Teacher Confidence Tips	Some pupils may have personal experience with vaping. Be empathetic, maintain a non-judgemental tone and have support resources ready. Running through the starter quiz and discussion questions beforehand can boost your confidence in facilitating the lesson smoothly. Emphasise healthy choices and alternatives to vaping, helping pupils feel empowered rather than scared.

KS3 Lesson 5

Lesson Title	Understanding Peer Pressure	**Key Stage**	3
		Lesson Length	50 minutes
Lesson Objectives			
• Identify what peer pressure is and recognise common situations where it occurs. • Explain the effects of peer pressure on decision-making, especially related to harmful substances. • Demonstrate effective strategies to resist peer pressure through role-play scenarios. • Reflect on personal experiences or thoughts about peer pressure and how to handle it positively.			

<table>
<tr><td>Resources Needed</td><td><ul><li>Printed or digital role-play scenario cards</li><li>Pens and paper or exercise books</li><li>A whiteboard or flip chart and markers</li><li>Large room or area</li></ul></td><td>Key Vocabulary</td><td>Peer pressure, influence, substance, harmful, consequences, assertive, refusal skills, risk, addiction, decision-making, support system, boundaries</td></tr>
<tr><td>Starter Activity (10 minutes)</td><td colspan="3">Review the learner agreement as a class.
Ask pupils to spend 1–2 minutes thinking silently about these questions:<ul><li>What is peer pressure?</li><li>Can you give an example of a situation where someone might feel pressured by their friends to do something they don't want to?</li></ul>Have pupils turn to a partner and share their thoughts and examples. Give them 1–2 minutes to discuss. Encourage them to listen carefully and add to each other's ideas.
Bring the class back together and ask a few pairs to share their examples aloud. Highlight common themes and briefly explain that peer pressure can be both direct and indirect, and sometimes it relates to making choices about substances.
If you have time, you could also ask the question:
'How does social media influence young people's choices about substances like vaping, alcohol or drugs?'
Ask pupils to first think about their answer individually for 1–2 minutes, then discuss their ideas with a partner. Finally, bring the whole class together to share key points and encourage a brief group discussion on the impact of social media as a form of peer pressure.</td></tr>
</table>

<table>
<tr><td>Main Activity (30 minutes)</td><td>Divide the class into small groups of 3–4 pupils. Tell them that each group will create a short role play showing a realistic situation where someone is facing peer pressure to use harmful substances (such as alcohol, vaping or cannabis).

Let pupils know they don't have to act if they're uncomfortable. Instead, they can

• Watch and give feedback to others.
• Draw a comic strip showing how someone could respond.
• Write out a short dialogue instead of performing it.

Give each group a different peer pressure scenario to work with (KS3 Lesson 5 Resource 1). Use everyday situations that pupils can relate to. For example,

• Being offered a vape at a party.
• Friends encouraging someone to drink energy drinks before a sports game.
• Being teased for not drinking alcohol at a social event.

Next, ask groups to talk about their scenario, choose roles and practise acting it out. Remind them to show how the person being pressured could respond in either a positive or negative way.

Each group performs their role play (2–3 minutes per group). After each performance, lead a short class discussion on what happened:

• How did the person deal with the pressure?
• What worked well?
• What could they have done differently?

Key points that should be emphasised are
• How to say no confidently.
• The importance of making your own decisions.
• How supportive friends can make a difference.</td></tr>
<tr><td>Plenary</td><td>Ask pupils to spend 3 minutes writing down one thing they learned about peer pressure and one strategy they would use to resist it.

Have pupils pair up and share their reflections for 3 minutes.

Facilitate a whole-class discussion for 4 minutes where a few volunteers share their thoughts.

Summarise key points and reinforce the message that it's okay to make their own choices and real friends will respect those choices.</td></tr>
</table>

<table>
<tr><td>Assessment Ideas</td><td colspan="3">Starter activity
Assess pupils' baseline understanding by listening to and noting their answers to the initial questions.

Main Activity
Observe how pupils use strategies to handle peer pressure in realistic situations during their role-plays, paying attention to their communication skills and problem-solving approaches. During the whole-class discussion, listen carefully to their contributions to assess their understanding of the concepts and their ability to express ideas clearly.

Plenary
Review pupils' written reflections to assess what they've learned and their ability to identify personal strategies.</td></tr>
<tr><td rowspan="2">Signposting and Support</td><td rowspan="2"><u>Website Support</u>
Talk to Frank: Information on drugs including vaping and how to get help.

www.talktofrank.com

Phone: 0300 123 6600

YoungMinds: Support for mental health, which can be linked to addiction and stress.

www.youngminds.org.uk</td><td>Cross-Topic Links</td><td>Science (biology), citizenship, English, drama</td></tr>
<tr><td>Teacher Confidence Tips</td><td>Before the lesson, read through or even practice the role-play examples yourself. This helps you feel comfortable managing group dynamics, prompts and how to model assertive responses pupils might use in real life.

At the start, explain that this is a judgement-free lesson where everyone is respected. Making pupils feel safe encourages honest conversation.</td></tr>
</table>

KS3 Lesson 6

<table>
<tr><td>Lesson Title</td><td>Debate: Is Social Media as Harmful as Drugs and Alcohol for Mental Health?</td><td>Key Stage
Lesson Length</td><td>3
50 minutes</td></tr>
<tr><td colspan="4">Lesson Objectives</td></tr>
<tr><td colspan="4">• Understand what dopamine is and explain its role in reward-seeking behaviours.
• Identify and compare the potential impacts of social media, drugs and alcohol on young people's mental health.
• Develop and express arguments in a structured debate, using evidence and examples.
• Develop confidence in speaking, listening and critical thinking.</td></tr>
<tr><td>Resources Needed</td><td>• Access to YouTube
• Debate prompt questions
• Fact sheets or articles on the impact of social media on mental health and the effects of drugs and alcohol on the brain
• Laptops for group research (optional)</td><td>Key Vocabulary</td><td>Dopamine, addiction, mental health, social media, neurotransmitter, reward system, impulse control, debate, rebuttal, opening statement, counter-argument</td></tr>
<tr><td>Starter Activity (10 minutes)</td><td colspan="3">Review the learner agreement as a class.
As pupils enter, have the following question written on the board:
'What is dopamine, and what do you think it does in your brain and body?'
Hand out sticky notes or small slips of paper. Ask pupils to take 2–3 minutes to write their thoughts. Remind them there are no wrong answers. This is just to see what they already know.
While they're writing, circulate the room to check for engagement and early misconceptions (e.g. 'dopamine is always bad').
Ask a few volunteers to read theirs aloud or anonymously collect responses and read a few out to the class.
Briefly summarise key correct ideas (e.g. 'Dopamine is a chemical in your brain that makes you feel good, like a reward signal') but avoid over-explaining at this point. The goal is to revisit this concept later in the lesson.</td></tr>
</table>

<table>
<tr>
<td>Main Activity (30 minutes)</td>
<td>Watch & Debate: Is Social Media as Harmful as Drugs and Alcohol for Mental Health?
Begin by playing one of the following videos on YouTube (or another reputable source on addiction and social media's impact):
• Video 1: How Social Media Affects the Brain
https://youtu.be/rooEBjZWpDc?si=rZm767WYl-TnItMF
• Video 2: The Science of Social Media Addiction
https://www.youtube.com/watch?v=c7fT9U3Q2-o&t=29s
Before watching the video, ask pupils to take notes on key points, especially any mention of dopamine, mental health, addiction or comparison with substance use. Explain that this will help them form evidence-based arguments later in the lesson.
Next, divide the class into two teams:
• Team A: Argues that social media is just as harmful as drugs and alcohol.
• Team B: Argues that social media is less harmful than drugs and alcohol.
Pupils can choose their side or be assigned a team at random to promote critical thinking and balanced engagement.
Distribute a prompt sheet with (KS3 Lesson 5 Resource 1) and a debate planning sheet with (KS3 Lesson 5 Resource 2) to each team.
Here are the questions on the prompt sheet:
• What is dopamine and how does it relate to addiction?
• What are the known mental health effects of social media?
• How do drugs and alcohol affect mental health?
• Can social media be used in healthy ways?
Pupils should use video notes, prior knowledge and class resources to prepare their argument.
Take a minute to read through the prompt sheet (KS3 Lesson 5 Resource 1) as a class. This resource includes key questions to help the pupils to explore the topic from different angles, such as how dopamine relates to addiction, the mental health impact of social media and the effects of drugs and alcohol. Use this as a starting point for discussion.
Then, get them to begin using the debate planning sheet (KS3 Lesson 5 Resource 2) to organise their ideas. This template will help them to structure their argument by
• Using evidence or examples that support their side.
• Anticipating what the other team might say and how they will respond.
• Planning who will say what during the debate so everyone has a role.</td>
</tr>
</table>

	Support inclusion by providing sentence starters, keyword cards or simplified fact sheets for pupils who need scaffolding (e.g. EAL or SEND learners). Encourage collaboration within teams. Use this clear structure to keep the debate focused and fair: • **Opening statements**: 1 minute per team. • **Alternating arguments**: 2 minutes per team (each team goes twice). • **Cross-examination**: Each team asks the other one question and allows time for a response (2 minutes per team). • **Closing statements**: 1 minute per team. • **Audience vote**: Non-speaking pupils vote for the most convincing side. If everyone speaks, you may cast the final vote.
Plenary (10 minutes)	Ask pupils to write a short written reflection in response to these questions: • What did you learn about the impact of dopamine on mental health? • Has this changed how you think about social media or substances like alcohol and drugs? Conclude the lesson by briefly summarising the key points discussed during the session, including the impact of social media and drugs/alcohol on mental health and dopamine release. Reinforce the importance of understanding these effects and encourage pupils to consider how this knowledge applies to their own lives. Keep the summary concise and use simple language to ensure clarity.
Assessment Ideas	**Starter Activity** Assess pupils' ability to extract key ideas about the effects of social media and substance use by reviewing their notes taken during the video(s) and their responses to discussion prompts. Also evaluate how well they begin to make connections between dopamine, mental health, and addiction. **Main Activity** During group preparation and the structured debate, observe how effectively pupils collaborate to build a case using facts and reasoning, while communicating clearly, respectfully, and presenting coherent arguments. Assess their understanding and articulation of mental health risks, addictive behaviours, and the role of social media. Look for evidence of empathy, curiosity, or a shift in viewpoint based on new information. Use targeted questioning, especially during cross-examination, to challenge assumptions and deepen thinking. For pupils not speaking in the debate, evaluate their contributions through written notes, support roles such as summarising or poster design, or through observational checklists.

<table>
<tr><td></td><td colspan="3">Plenary
Use the audience vote to gauge the persuasive impact of the debate and identify which arguments resonated most. Ask pupils to complete a short written reflection on the most convincing point they heard and why. Review these reflections to assess their critical engagement, understanding of the topic, and any lingering misconceptions. Use this insight to inform planning for follow-up lessons or pastoral discussions on digital well-being.</td></tr>
<tr><td rowspan="2">Signposting and Support</td><td rowspan="2"><u>Website Support</u>
YoungMinds: Supports young people's mental health with advice and helplines.
www.youngminds.org.uk
Kooth: Online mental health support platform for young people.
www.kooth.com</td><td>Cross-Topic Links</td><td>Science (biology), citizenship, English/literacy, media studies, politics</td></tr>
<tr><td>Teacher Confidence Tips</td><td>Review key facts about dopamine, addiction and mental health beforehand so you can confidently clarify any pupil questions and guide discussions effectively.
Create a safe space where pupils feel comfortable sharing different opinions. Remind yourself that diverse views enrich the debate and it is ok if you don't have all the answers.
Rely on clear debate rules and time limits to manage the discussion. This will help maintain focus, ensure all voices are heard and boost your confidence in handling lively conversations.</td></tr>
</table>

4 KS4: Lesson Plans

KS4 Lesson 1

Lesson Title	Understanding the Effects of Common Substances	Key Stage	4
		Lesson Length	50 minutes
Lesson Objectives			
• Share existing knowledge about common substances and their effects. • Explain how different substances impact the body and mind. • Describe the short-term and long-term risks associated with substance use. • Demonstrate understanding to make informed decisions about substance use.			
Resources Needed	• Quiz sheets or digital quiz platform • Fact sheets or handouts • Whiteboard and markers, pens and paper, interactive tools like Kahoot or Mentimeter (optional)	**Key Vocabulary**	Substances, effects, addiction, physical health, mental health, dependency, withdrawal, risk factors, prevention, coping strategies, peer pressure, self-esteem
Creating Learner Agreement	Begin the lesson by establishing a positive and respectful classroom environment through the creation of a learner agreement. This sets clear expectations for behaviour, participation and respect, which helps all pupils feel safe and engaged. Briefly explain to pupils that the learner agreement is a set of shared rules everyone agrees to follow during the lesson (and ideally, throughout the series). Emphasise that this helps create a respectful space where everyone can learn and express their views safely. Invite pupils to contribute their ideas about what makes a good learning environment. Prompt with questions like • What behaviours help us learn best? • How can we respect each other's opinions? • What should we do if someone is disruptive?		

DOI: 10.4324/9781003608998-4

<table>
<tr><td></td><td>As pupils suggest behaviours, write these on the board or a visible flipchart. These might include
• Listen when others are speaking.
• Respect different opinions.
• Stay on task and participate.
• Use appropriate language.
• Keep phones away unless instructed (if applicable).
Refer to this agreement at the start of every lesson to reinforce expectations.</td></tr>
<tr><td>Starter Activity (10 minutes)</td><td>Briefly explain that today's lesson will focus on the effects of commonly used substances like alcohol, tobacco and cannabis.
Let them know that you'll start with a short quiz to find out what they already know. Emphasise that this is not a test, just a way to get them thinking and talking.
Hand out a printed quiz sheet (KS4 Lesson 1 Resource 1) or display questions on the board/projector.
If using mini whiteboards or digital devices, instruct pupils to prepare them.
Explain that they will answer each question independently. Give pupils time to answer each of the five multiple choice questions quietly and individually. Encourage them to answer all questions, even if unsure.
Go through the correct answers as a class. Use this moment to briefly clarify any misconceptions or prompt short discussions.
• What do you notice about which substances are legal versus illegal?
• Which of these substances are most familiar to young people and why?
Briefly summarise key correct ideas (e.g. 'Dopamine is a chemical in your brain that makes you feel good, like a reward signal'), but avoid over-explaining at this point. The goal is to revisit this concept later in the lesson.</td></tr>
<tr><td>Main Activity (30 minutes)</td><td>This activity helps pupils understand the short and long-term effects of commonly used substances, including alcohol, nicotine, cannabis, energy drinks and prescription medications. It also builds discussion around misconceptions and peer/media influence.
Before the lesson, prepare two sets of cards or printed sheets using KS4 Lesson 1 Resource 2:
• Substance cards: Include substances such as alcohol, nicotine, cannabis, energy drinks and prescription drugs.
• Effect cards: Include physical, emotional and social effects such as addiction, anxiety, liver damage, peer pressure, sleep disruption, impaired judgement and lung damage.</td></tr>
</table>

	Organise pupils into small groups of 3–4. Hand out one full set of substance cards and one full set of effect cards to each group. Also give them access to a fact sheet that outlines basic information about each substance. Pupils work together to discuss and match each substance to any relevant effects, noting that one substance may have multiple effects and some effects may apply to more than one substance. Encourage pupils to talk through their reasoning and use the fact sheet if unsure. Ask them to note down any surprises or misconceptions they uncover during the task. For example, the fact that energy drinks can cause sleep disruption or anxiety may surprise some. Display or read aloud the following discussion questions, and ask each group to reflect: • Which substances had affects you didn't expect? • Why do you think some effects are underestimated or misunderstood by young people? • How might peer pressure, social media or advertising influence someone's choices or beliefs about these substances? Circulate during discussions, listening in to conversations and offering prompts where needed. Use this time to informally assess pupils' understanding. Invite each group to share one key insight, surprising link or misconception they uncovered. This helps to consolidate learning across the class. Use this sharing time to • Clarify or correct any inaccurate ideas. • Emphasise key takeaways (e.g. not all harmful substances are illegal, or that legal substances like alcohol and nicotine still carry significant long-term risks). • Reinforce the message that understanding effects helps empower informed and confident decision-making.
Plenary (10 minutes)	Ask each pupil to write a short response (2–3 sentences) to the question: 'What is one new thing you learned today about the effects of substances, and why do you think it is important?' Collect these at the end of the lesson to assess understanding and engagement. Conduct a rapid-fire multiple-choice quiz using 3–5 questions from the earlier quiz you created. • You can do this orally, with a show of hands, or using quiz apps/tools if available. • Give immediate feedback to reinforce learning and clarify misconceptions.

<table>
<tr>
<td>**Assessment Ideas**</td>
<td colspan="3">**Starter Activity**
Use pupils' responses to the initial multiple-choice quiz to assess their prior knowledge of commonly used substances and their effects. Look for gaps or misconceptions (e.g. underestimating risks of legal substances like alcohol or energy drinks). This provides a baseline for measuring progress later in the lesson.
Main Activity
Observe how pupils engage in the substance-effect matching activity and group discussion. Listen for accurate identification of short- and long-term effects, the ability to explain reasoning using facts or prior knowledge and any misconceptions or surprising beliefs that may need addressing. Review any written notes or completed worksheets. These provide useful evidence of how pupils are processing and applying information
Plenary
Use the short exit ticket or written reflection to assess individual understanding. Look out for clarity in describing one key fact they learned, insight into how their thinking has changed or why and signs of critical thinking or personal connection to the topic.</td>
</tr>
<tr>
<td rowspan="2">**Signposting and Support**</td>
<td rowspan="2">**Website Support**
Talk to Frank: Honest and accessible information about drugs, including risks and where to seek support.
www.talktofrank.com
Phone: 0300 123 6600
YoungMinds: Mental health charity for young people. Includes information on stress, anxiety, depression and where to get help.
www.youngminds.org.uk
Kooth: Online mental health support platform for young people.
www.kooth.com
The Mix: Support for under-25s covering topics like drugs, mental health, relationships and self-care.
www.themix.org.uk</td>
<td>**Cross-Topic Links**</td>
<td>Science (biology), citizenship, English/ communication</td>
</tr>
<tr>
<td>**Teacher Confidence Tips**</td>
<td>Knowing your material inside and out builds confidence in delivering it smoothly.
Rehearse handling sensitive topics and possible pupil reactions to feel ready for anything.
After lessons, note what went well to remind yourself of your effectiveness and progress.
Keep informed on current trends and facts about substance use to maintain credibility and relevance.</td>
</tr>
</table>

KS4 Lesson 2

<table>
<tr><td>Lesson Title</td><td>Managing Peer/Media Influence and Self-Esteem</td><td>Key Stage</td><td>4</td></tr>
<tr><td></td><td></td><td>Lesson Length</td><td>50 minutes</td></tr>
<tr><td colspan="4">Lesson Objectives</td></tr>
<tr><td colspan="4">• Identify how peer pressure and media influence can affect self-esteem and decision-making.
• Describe strategies to manage negative peer or media influence in real-life situations.
• Reflect on how social media and friendships shape self-image and confidence.
• Demonstrate ways to respond assertively when feeling pressured by others.</td></tr>
<tr><td>Resources Needed</td><td>• Printed scenario cards for starter activity
• 'Sort the Scenarios' worksheet or whiteboards
• Printed scenario cards (10–12) for main activity
• Printed worksheets for group responses
• Post-it notes</td><td>Key Vocabulary</td><td>Peer pressure, media influence, self-esteem, confidence, assertiveness, boundaries, influencer, pressure, risk-taking, coping strategy</td></tr>
<tr><td>Starter Activity (10 minutes)</td><td colspan="3">Review the learner agreement as a class.

This starter activity will activate prior knowledge and get pupils thinking critically about how peer pressure and media can affect self-esteem.

Prepare slips of paper or a digital slide with these short scenarios (KS4 Lesson 2 Resource 1).
• Your friend dares you to vape at lunch, saying everyone's doing it.
• An influencer posts a photo of a 'perfect' body and says, 'No excuses!'
• A classmate suggests skipping class to hang out, saying it's no big deal.
• Your teacher pressures you to fight someone to prove you're brave (clearly unrealistic).

In pairs or small groups, pupils must sort each scenario into
• Realistic pressure/influence.
• Exaggerated or unlikely.
• Unsure.

After 3–4 minutes, have a whole-class discussion to clarify which are most common in real life, and what makes a scenario realistic.</td></tr>
</table>

<table>
<tr>
<td>Main Activity</td>
<td>
Preparation (before the lesson)
Print and cut out the scenario cards (KS4 Lesson 2 Resource 2) that describe short, age-appropriate and realistic examples of peer or media pressure. Number each card clearly so groups can refer to them easily during discussion. Example scenarios might include
• A friend dares you to vape at a party.
• You feel bad after seeing filtered selfies online.
• An influencer promotes a 'magic' weight-loss tea.
• Your mates make fun of someone who doesn't drink.
• You see a TikTok challenge encouraging risky behaviour.
• Someone tells you you're boring if you don't take something 'just once.'
Introduce the activity by asking the question:
'What does it mean to be influenced by others?'
Invite a few responses. Use these to explore key definitions as a class:
• Peer pressure: The influence friends or acquaintances can have on your decisions.
• Media influence: The way social media, influencers and celebrities can shape how we think or act.
• Self-esteem: How we see and value ourselves.
Display or write these terms and definitions clearly on the board to support all learners and provide a shared vocabulary for the task.
Next, divide the class into small groups of 3–4 pupils. Give each group 2–3 scenario cards and a worksheet with the following discussion prompts:
• What's happening in this scenario?
• How could this situation make someone feel?
• What's a confident or positive way to respond?
Encourage pupils to discuss openly, draw from their own experiences or previous PSHE lessons, and consider both emotional and social consequences. Groups should write one confident, assertive response for each card (e.g. what they might say or do in that situation).
Circulate between groups to listen in, prompt deeper thinking and challenge surface-level responses. Ask open-ended questions such as
• Why might someone feel pressured here?
• What makes this a hard situation to navigate?
• What would you want a friend to say or do in this moment?
</td>
</tr>
</table>

	This is a good moment to highlight that confident responses don't have to be confrontational. Suggest that assertiveness, humour, deflection and boundary-setting are all valid. Ask each group to read out one scenario and their agreed confident response. Encourage others to listen respectfully and offer additional ideas. Create a quick class display of 'Confident Comebacks' by writing the best responses on the board or collecting them for a wall resource. This activity helps to normalise assertiveness and gives pupils practical, peer-generated tools for resisting pressure in real-life situations.
Plenary (10 minutes)	Distribute a Post-it note or index card to each pupil. Ask them to quietly write down the following: • One thing I've learned today about peer or media pressure is . . . • I can respond to it by . . . After 2–3 minutes of writing time, invite a few pupils to share what they've written (voluntarily only). You might say: 'Would anyone like to share something they're taking away from today's lesson?' Acknowledge responses positively. Ask pupils to stick their notes on a 'Learning Wall' or hand them in as they leave. This gives you informal assessment data and closes the lesson reflectively.
Assessment Ideas	**Starter Activity** Gauge pupils' baseline understanding of peer/media influence by listening to their reasoning and choices during scenario-based discussions. **Main Activity** Assess how well pupils identify types of influence and demonstrate strategies for resisting pressure or boosting self-esteem through group responses. **Plenary** Use the short written reflection ('One thing I've learned today about peer or media pressure . . .') to assess individual learning and identify key takeaways or misconceptions.

<table>
<tr>
<td rowspan="2">Signposting and Support</td>
<td rowspan="2"><u>Website Support</u>
YoungMinds: Excellent mental health resources, including tips on handling peer pressure, social media anxiety and building confidence.
www.youngminds.org.uk
Kooth: Online mental health support platform for young people.
www.kooth.com
<u>School Support</u>
School counsellor or pastoral lead: Pupils struggling with confidence, peer pressure or social media-related stress can be referred for one-to-one support or group sessions.
Well-being ambassadors or peer mentoring programmes: Encourage pupils to connect with trained peers who promote positive self-esteem and help others build resilience.
Designated safeguarding lead (DSL): In cases where peer or media influence causes harm or distress, pupils should know they can report concerns to the DSL confidentially.
Pastoral support team: Point out that tutors and pastoral staff are there to provide guidance and support in managing peer pressure or self-esteem issues.
Peer mentoring or well-being groups: Mention any school-run clubs or groups focused on health, well-being or positive choices, where pupils can talk and get advice.</td>
<td>Cross-Topic Links</td>
<td>Science (biology), citizenship,
English/literacy, media studies, personal safety</td>
</tr>
<tr>
<td>Teacher Confidence Tips</td>
<td>Bring in current social media trends or popular adverts to make the lesson relatable and spark genuine interest.
Create a safe space where pupils feel comfortable sharing their thoughts without judgement to boost engagement.
Keep informed on current trends and facts about substance use to maintain credibility and relevance.
Smiling, making eye contact and speaking clearly can build rapport and make you feel more confident.</td>
</tr>
</table>

KS4 Lesson 3

<table>
<tr><td rowspan="2">Lesson Title</td><td rowspan="2">Psychological Reasons for Taking Drugs and Healthy Coping Strategies</td><td>Key Stage</td><td>4</td></tr>
<tr><td>Lesson Length</td><td>50 minutes</td></tr>
<tr><td colspan="4">Lesson Objectives</td></tr>
<tr><td colspan="4">• Describe common psychological reasons why some people might turn to substances.
• Identify the difference between healthy and unhealthy coping strategies.
• Evaluate the effectiveness of different coping methods in stressful or emotional situations.
• Reflect on methods of coping and consider alternatives.</td></tr>
<tr><td>Resources Needed</td><td>• Printed case studies
• Worksheet or reflection templates
• PowerPoint or visual aid presentation
• Post-it notes or slips of paper
• Whiteboard or flip chart</td><td>Key Vocabulary</td><td>Addiction, mental health, coping strategies, triggers, stress, anxiety, depression, peer influence, self-medication, risk factors, resilience, emotional regulation, support networks, substance misuse</td></tr>
<tr><td>Starter Activity</td><td colspan="3">Review the learner agreement as a class.
Begin by saying,
Today we're exploring why some people might turn to drugs, alcohol or other substances. Often, it's not just about the substance, it's about what someone is trying to manage or escape from. Let's start by thinking about reasons why that might happen.
On the board, display some or all of these sentence starters to get pupils to complete.
• Someone might drink alcohol to . . .
• A person might take drugs because . . .
• If someone is feeling overwhelmed, they might . . .
• When people feel anxious or stressed, they sometimes . . .
• A teenager might struggle to cope when . . .
• Someone might not know how to ask for help if . . .</td></tr>
</table>

<table>
<tr><td></td><td>Think-Pair-Share
Pupils reflect on one or two prompts, then pair up and share thoughts. Gather 2–3 responses per prompt in a class discussion.
Ask the pupils
• What patterns do you notice?
• Were any reasons surprising?
• How many of these are linked to emotions or mental health?</td></tr>
<tr><td>Main Activity</td><td>Introduce the task with a short explanation to frame the learning intention. You might say:

We've just explored some of the emotional and psychological reasons why someone might turn to substances. Now you're going to apply that learning to real-life situations. Each group will now work through a scenario involving a young person dealing with stress, anxiety or pressure, and you'll think about what's going on, what risks are involved and what healthier coping responses could look like.

Remind pupils there are no 'perfect' answers. This is about developing understanding, not judgement.

Provide case studies (KS4 Lesson 3 Resource 1):
• Scenario 1: Aiden is struggling with exam pressure. He says drinking at parties helps him 'switch off.'
• Scenario 2: Sophie feels isolated at school. Her online friend offers her pills that 'help you feel happy.'
• Scenario 3: Liam's parents argue constantly. He starts vaping to feel calmer.
• Scenario 4: Priya feels overwhelmed balancing school and caring for her younger sibling. She skips meals and sleeps a lot to escape.

Place pupils into pairs or groups of 3–4 and give each group 1–2 scenarios (printed or digital). Provide each group with the analysis framework, either as a handout or on the board (KS4 Lesson 3 Resource 2).
• What emotion/s is the person experiencing?
• What substance or behaviour are they turning to?
• Why do you think they chose that coping strategy?
• What are the short- and long-term consequences?
• What healthier coping strategies could they use instead?
• How could a friend or trusted adult help?

Encourage pupils to make bullet-point notes and focus on understanding the emotional drivers behind behaviour, rather than judging the choices made.</td></tr>
</table>

	Support groups by circulating, asking open-ended questions such as • What might have influenced their choice? • How do you think they felt before, during and after? Each group briefly presents their scenario and 1–2 key insights to the rest of the class. You can use a whiteboard or flipchart to summarise common themes (e.g. stress, loneliness, family pressure). Prompt reflection and class discussion with questions like: • Do you think they made that choice because they lacked support? • What might have helped them choose differently? • Have you seen or heard of similar situations in media or in life? This phase reinforces the message that substance use often has emotional roots, and that building awareness, empathy and alternatives is essential for harm reduction and personal resilience. This activity supports PSHE learning by bridging emotional understanding and real-world decision-making, helping pupils develop both empathy and practical coping tools they can carry forward.
Plenary (10 minutes)	Ask pupils to reflect on the lesson and write short answers to the following: • What is one healthy coping strategy you learned about today? • In what kind of situation might it help you or someone else? • What would you say to a friend who is struggling and considering substance use to cope? You can write these questions on the board or present them on a slide. Invite a few pupils to share their answers voluntarily. Then collect the reflections as they leave or ask pupils to place them in a 'reflection box' near the door. End the activity by saying something like, Substances may seem like a solution to emotional stress, but there are safer, healthier ways to cope. Keep today's strategies in mind for yourself and to support others.
Assessment Ideas	**Starter Activity** Use pupil responses during the initial scenario-based discussion ('Why might someone turn to drugs in a stressful situation?') to assess their baseline understanding of emotional stress and coping behaviours. Look for evidence of empathy, emotional insight or common misconceptions. Gauge how confidently pupils can connect real-life pressures with behaviour and whether they show awareness of alternative responses.

<table>
<tr>
<td></td>
<td colspan="3">Main Activity
Observe how pupils engage with their group's scenario analysis. Assess their ability to identify and explain unhealthy versus healthy coping strategies, and how well they understand the emotional triggers behind each choice. Listen for depth of reasoning, respectful peer discussion and teamwork. Use open-ended questioning to encourage deeper thinking (e.g. 'Why might someone feel this is their only option?' or 'How realistic is that alternative in the real world?'). Note which pupils are able to evaluate strategies critically and which may need further support in developing emotional literacy.
Plenary
Review pupils' written reflections to assess their ability to apply learning to real-life contexts. Look for thoughtful identification of healthier coping methods and an ability to reflect personally or empathetically on the scenarios. Strong responses will show personal insight, practical awareness and an ability to think beyond the lesson. These reflections can also serve as a useful tool for identifying pupils who may benefit from additional follow-up or pastoral check-in.</td>
</tr>
<tr>
<td rowspan="2">Signposting and Support</td>
<td rowspan="2"><u>Website Support</u>
YoungMinds: Excellent mental health resources, including tips on handling peer pressure, social media anxiety and building confidence.
www.youngminds.org.uk
Kooth: Online mental health support platform for young people.
www.kooth.com
<u>School Support</u>
Well-being ambassadors or peer mentoring programmes: Encourage pupils to connect with trained peers who promote positive self-esteem and help others build resilience.
Pastoral support team: Point out that tutors and pastoral staff are there to provide guidance and support in managing peer pressure or self-esteem issues.</td>
<td>Cross-Topic Links</td>
<td>Science (biology), mental health, citizenship, English/literacy, sociology</td>
</tr>
<tr>
<td>Teacher Confidence Tips</td>
<td>If sensitive topics arise (e.g. trauma, addiction, mental health struggles), be prepared to remind pupils of safeguarding boundaries.
Reassure them that it's okay to speak privately after the session and know the referral routes to your school's pastoral team or counsellor.</td>
</tr>
</table>

			Instead of labelling behaviours as 'bad,' encourage discussion around helpful versus unhelpful strategies. This avoids judgement and helps you create a more open, supportive classroom space which encourages honest reflection.

KS4 Lesson 4

<table>
<tr><td rowspan="2">Lesson Title</td><td rowspan="2">Substance Use and Relationships</td><td>Key Stage</td><td>4</td></tr>
<tr><td>Lesson Length</td><td>50 minutes</td></tr>
<tr><td colspan="4">Lesson Objectives</td></tr>
<tr><td colspan="4">• Understand how substance use can affect personal relationships, including with family, friends and romantic partners.
• Identify the signs of strained or toxic relationships linked to substance misuse.
• Explore the emotional, social and behavioural consequences of substance use on communication and trust.
• Evaluate strategies for maintaining healthy relationships and offering or seeking support when substance use is involved.</td></tr>
<tr><td>Resources Needed</td><td>• Printed or digital copies of relationship case study scenarios
• Response sheet
• A3 paper or whiteboards for group mind mapping
• Pens or markers
• Paper or exercise books</td><td>Key Vocabulary</td><td>Substance use, dependency, co-dependency, trust, boundaries, conflict, communication, emotional impact, co-dependency, peer influence, respect, support systems</td></tr>
<tr><td>Starter Activity (10 minutes)</td><td colspan="3">Review the learner agreement as a class.
On mini whiteboards or in notebooks, ask pupils to quickly list five different types of relationships they have in their life (e.g. friend, parent/carer, sibling, romantic partner, teacher, coach).
In pairs, pupils pick two from their list and briefly discuss the following prompt:
'What makes this relationship strong or healthy?'
Encourage key words like trust, respect, communication, boundaries and honesty.
Record pupil suggestions on the board under 'What healthy relationships need.'
Show the final reflection question:
'What could put these things at risk?'
This sets the stage for introducing how substances might affect these elements.</td></tr>
</table>

	'What might happen to our relationships if substance use starts to influence behaviour, communication or trust?' Encourage pupils to think critically and consider how changes caused by alcohol, drugs or dependency can affect emotions, reliability and personal boundaries. Let pupils briefly share their thoughts before introducing the main activity.
Main Activity (30 minutes)	Now split the class into small groups of 3–4 pupils. Assign each group a Response Sheet (**KS4 Lesson 4 Resource 2**) with guiding questions for each case study: 1. What is happening in this situation? 2. How is the relationship being affected? 3. What advice or healthy support could help this person or their relationship? Pupils will rotate through the stations in carousel format, spending 7–8 minutes at each one. At each station, they will • Read the case study together. • Discuss the scenario, focusing on emotions, consequences and possible responses. • Complete the corresponding section of their response sheet. As pupils work, circulate around the room to support and extend thinking. Use open-ended questions such as • How do you think this person might justify their behaviour? • Is the friend/family member reacting fairly? • What boundaries or communication might help this relationship recover? • How does peer influence show up in this scenario? After all rotations are complete, gather the class for a debrief. Ask each group to share the case study they found most thought-provoking or difficult and explain: • What made it stand out? • What support strategies did they come up with? Use this time to reinforce the importance of empathy, communication and recognising how substance use can create ripple effects in relationships. **Case Study Examples** • **Case A**: A teen hides vaping from their best friend, who finds out and feels betrayed. • **Case B**: Someone begins drinking heavily on weekends and starts missing time with family.

<table>
<tr><td></td><td colspan="3">• Case C: A romantic partner feels pressure to try weed to stay connected.
• Case D: A pupil starts skipping school to hang with a group that uses substances.
Encourage pupils to reflect not only on the behaviours, but also on the relational consequences and what healthy choices or support could look like in real life.</td></tr>
<tr><td>Plenary</td><td colspan="3">Hand out small slips of paper to each pupil
Ask pupils to imagine a friend is struggling with stress and considering turning to substances (alcohol, vaping, etc.) to cope.
Task: Write a short piece of advice to this friend, including
• One healthy coping strategy they've learned today.
• One reason why turning to substances is not the best choice.
Encourage them to be empathetic, realistic and supportive in their response.</td></tr>
<tr><td>Assessment Ideas</td><td colspan="3">Starter Activity
Use pupil responses in the group discussion or sorting task to gauge prior understanding of why people turn to substances and what healthy coping strategies they already know.
Main Activity
Observe pupils' group discussions or role plays to assess how well they can identify, explain and evaluate coping strategies. Use open-ended questions to prompt deeper thinking.
Plenary
Review pupils' written advice to assess their understanding of psychological motivations and their ability to suggest realistic, healthy alternatives.</td></tr>
<tr><td rowspan="2">Signposting and Support</td><td rowspan="2"><u>Website Support</u>
YoungMinds: Excellent mental health resources, including tips on handling peer pressure, social media anxiety and building confidence.
www.youngminds.org.uk
Kooth: Online mental health support platform for young people.
www.kooth.com</td><td>Cross-Topic Links</td><td>Science (biology), psychology, religious education, citizenship, English/ literacy, sociology, relationships, education</td></tr>
<tr><td>Teacher Confidence Tips</td><td>Prepare relatable, age-appropriate scenarios that reflect real-life relationship dynamics affected by substance use (e.g. tension in friendships or family breakdown).</td></tr>
</table>

	Talk to Frank: Honest and accessible information about drugs, including risks and where to seek support. www.talktofrank.com Phone: 0300 123 6600 **School Support** **Pastoral support team**: Point out that tutors and pastoral staff are there to provide guidance and support in managing peer pressure or self-esteem issues.		This grounds the discussion and makes abstract ideas more tangible. This topic can hit close to home. Acknowledge that some pupils may have personal experience with substance misuse in their family or community. Offer opt-outs for sensitive tasks and remind pupils of available support.

KS4 Lesson 5

Lesson Title	Debate: Should There Be a Smoking Ban?	**Key Stage**	4
		Lesson Length	50 minutes
Lesson Objectives			
• Understand the main arguments for and against a smoking ban. • Use evidence to support my point of view in a debate. • Listen to and respond respectfully to opposing opinions. • Develop my skills in presenting clear and persuasive arguments.			
Resources Needed	• Whiteboard or flipchart • Timer or stopwatch • Debate Planning Sheet • Pens and paper • Access to online articles or fact sheets on smoking legislation and health effects to support pupil research • Reflection prompt sheet	**Key Vocabulary**	Ban, legislation, public health, second-hand smoke, addiction, harm reduction, prohibition, rights, personal freedom, economic impact, debate, argument, evidence, persuasion, counterargument, policy

<table>
<tr><td>Starter Activity</td><td>Review the learner agreement as a class.

Introduce the statement by writing or displaying it on the board:
'Smoking should be completely banned in the United Kingdom.'
Set up an opinion line. Label four points across the room:
• Strongly Agree
• Agree
• Disagree
• Strongly Disagree
Give the pupils 30 seconds to choose where they stand. Emphasise that there's no right or wrong answer.

Think–Pair–Share
• Ask pupils to briefly explain their reasoning to a peer near to them.
• Randomly pick 1–2 pupils from each group to share their views with the class.

Present 2–3 key statistics using a visual (slide/handout), e.g.
• 11.9 % of adults are smokers in the United Kingdom (ASH, 2021)
• £2.6 billion NHS costs linked to smoking (NHS Digital, 2023)

Ask: 'Now that you've seen some real-world stats, would anyone like to move?' Allow 1–2 minutes for movement and brief reflection.</td></tr>
<tr><td>Main Activity (30 minutes)</td><td>Introduce the Debate Topic (2 minutes)
Reintroduce the central question:

'Should smoking be completely banned in the United Kingdom?'

Clarify that this includes all tobacco products and could extend to vaping. Emphasise that the debate will help pupils explore multiple perspectives and build skills in persuasive speaking, critical thinking and evidence-based argument.

Divide the class by choosing one of the following approaches:

Option A: Allow pupils to choose the side they feel most strongly about.

Option B: Assign sides randomly to encourage flexible thinking and empathy for opposing views.

Optional: Within each team, assign roles such as speaker, researcher, note-taker and timekeeper. This helps pupils stay organised and engaged.

Preparation (5 minutes)
Give each team a handout or slide deck with key facts, statistics, expert quotes and balanced viewpoints, including sources that argue both for and against the ban. Highlight key vocabulary such as legislation, addiction, public health, rights, personal freedom and economic impact. Clarify any unfamiliar terms.</td></tr>
</table>

	Planning Arguments (8–10 minutes) Pupils work collaboratively to develop **2–3 strong arguments**, using evidence from the materials provided and debate planning sheet (**KS4 Lesson 5 Resource 1**). Encourage them to • Anticipate and address likely counterarguments. • Use **rhetorical devices** (e.g. rhetorical questions, emotive language, repetition) to strengthen their delivery. • Practise delivering key points clearly and persuasively. **Class Debate (10–15 minutes)** Follow a simple structure to keep the debate focused and fair: • **Opening statement**: 1 minute per team. • **Rebuttal round**: 1 minute per team. • **Open floor**: Allow the audience to ask questions or offer challenges. • **Closing remarks**: 30 seconds each side. Act as moderator and timekeeper, reminding pupils to use respectful language, listen actively, and avoid interruptions. Reinforce debate etiquette (e.g. 'I disagree because . . .' rather than 'You're wrong').
Plenary (10 minutes)	**Hand out the Reflection Prompt Sheet** (**KS4 Lesson 4 Resource 2**) **or display the questions on the board:** Ask pupils to respond to the following in their books or on a printed sheet: • What was your original opinion about banning smoking? • Did today's debate change your opinion? Why or why not? • What was one argument you heard that made you think differently? • What's your final view on whether smoking should be banned? Explain your reasoning. If time allows, invite 2–3 volunteers to read out a part of their reflection.
Assessment Ideas	**Starter Activity** Use initial class responses to the debate question ('Should smoking be completely banned in the United Kingdom?') to assess pupils' baseline attitudes and understanding of the issue. Listen for the use of relevant vocabulary and any misconceptions about public health, addiction or legislation. This will help identify which concepts may need reinforcing during the main activity.

<table>
<tr><td></td><td colspan="3">Main Activity
Observe group discussions as pupils prepare their arguments. Look for how well they use evidence from the provided materials and whether they can explain their points clearly. Assess their ability to work collaboratively, stay on task and apply critical thinking when considering counterarguments. During the debate, listen for confident delivery, appropriate use of persuasive language and structured reasoning. Take note of pupils who demonstrate empathy, flexibility and a willingness to engage with views different from their own.
Plenary (Post-Debate Reflection)
Use pupils' reflections on whether their opinions changed during the debate to assess their openness to new perspectives. Look for evidence of deeper understanding, improved reasoning and the ability to articulate why their thinking evolved. This provides insight into how well pupils can apply discussion and debate skills to real-world issues.</td></tr>
<tr><td rowspan="2">Signposting and Support</td><td rowspan="2"><u>Website Support</u>
NHS Smokefree: Offers facts about smoking, health risks, laws and quitting tips. A reliable resource for pupils to understand why smoking bans exist and their potential impacts.
www.nhs.uk/smokefree
Public Health England/Better Health Campaign: Offers educational materials about the risks of smoking and lifestyle improvements.
www.nhs.uk/better-health</td><td>Cross-Topic Links</td><td>Science (biology), politics, citizenship, English/literacy, media studies, history</td></tr>
<tr><td>Teacher Confidence Tips</td><td>A clear debate format (e.g. opening statements, rebuttals, closing points) will help pupils stay focused and give you control over the timing and flow. A visual timer or slide can help keep things moving.</td></tr>
</table>

	<u>School Support</u> **PSHE lead or pastoral team**: Can offer extra sessions or resources around decision-making, peer influence or related health concerns. **Pastoral support team**: Point out that tutors and pastoral staff are there to provide guidance and support in managing peer pressure or self-esteem issues.		Your role is to guide discussion, not influence the outcome. Remind yourself that your job is to encourage critical thinking, not to reach a consensus. For quieter pupils or if the debate wraps up early, have reflection tasks prepared (e.g. write a letter to an MP about your view on smoking laws). It ensures everyone stays meaningfully involved.

KS4 Lesson 6

Lesson Title	Legal and Social Consequences of Substance Abuse	**Key Stage**	4
		Lesson Length	50 minutes
Lesson Objectives			
• I can explain the legal consequences of using and supplying harmful substances. • I understand the social impact substance abuse can have on individuals, families and communities. • I can evaluate how breaking the law related to substances affects people's futures, including education and employment. • I can recognise the importance of making informed choices to avoid negative legal and social outcomes.			

<table>
<tr><td>Resources Needed</td><td>• Printed case studies
• Handouts summarising key laws and social impacts
• Interactive whiteboard (if using a presentation)
• Mini whiteboards and markers
• Response sheet</td><td>Key Vocabulary</td><td>Substance abuse, legal consequences, social consequences, addiction, law enforcement, penalty, prosecution, stigma, prevention</td></tr>
<tr><td>Starter Activity (10 minutes)</td><td colspan="3">Review the learner agreement as a class.

Display a real-world scenario (short and age-appropriate) involving a young person caught using, carrying or supplying substances (e.g. cannabis, nitrous oxide, prescription misuse).

Here is an example:

Jordan is 15 and was recently caught by school staff with a small amount of cannabis in his bag.
He says it was just for him and that he only uses it ‘now and then to chill out.’ He claims he didn’t plan to bring it to school. He just forgot it was in there. The school contacts his parents and informs the police.

In pairs, ask pupils to briefly discuss what they think the consequences could be for Jordan, legally and socially (e.g. criminal record, school exclusion, impact on job prospects and breakdown in friendships).

As a class, do a quick feedback session writing ideas on the board under two separate headings:

• Legal Consequences
• Social Consequences</td></tr>
<tr><td>Main Activity (30 minutes)</td><td colspan="3">Before the lesson, print out 4–6 different real-life or fictionalised case studies (KS4 Lesson Plan 6 Resource 1) along with handouts summarising key laws and social impacts These case studies involve teenagers or young adults experiencing consequences due to substance misuse. These will highlight a mix of

• Legal consequences: e.g. arrest, criminal record, fines, court involvement.
• Social consequences: e.g. loss of trust, school expulsion, breakdown of relationships, impact on future employment or university applications.

Each case study should be printed and cut out separately and placed at a clearly numbered station around the classroom. Consider including a mix of genders, backgrounds and substances to encourage broader discussion and engagement.</td></tr>
</table>

	Divide the class into small groups (3–4 pupils per group). Assign each group to a different station to start. Provide each group with a response sheet (**KS4 Lesson Plan 6 Resource 2**) containing guiding prompts such as • What happened in this scenario? • What were the short- and long-term legal/social consequences? • How did this affect the person's life, relationships or opportunities? • What alternative choices could have been made, and what might the outcomes have been? Allow each group 5 minutes per station to read the case study and complete the response sheet. After each time block, groups should rotate clockwise to the next station. Circulate around the room during this time, listening to discussions, clarifying details where needed and using open-ended questions to encourage deeper thinking (e.g. How might this consequence affect someone's future? or What could have changed the outcome?). Encourage pupils to compare the nature and severity of consequences across the different cases. Once all groups have visited every station, get together for a whole-class discussion. Ask each group to choose the case study they found most thought-provoking or impactful and explain why. Use this as a springboard to discuss common patterns, unexpected consequences and how decisions made in adolescence can have lasting effects. Draw links to pupils' own lives and choices, reinforcing the importance of critical thinking and peer influence in decision-making.
Plenary (10 minutes)	Say this to the pupils: Imagine a younger pupil at your school is starting to experiment with substances like alcohol, vape or cannabis. They think there's no real harm because 'everyone does it.' Based on what you've learned today, what would you say to help them understand the risks, especially the legal and social consequences? Ask pupils to write a short paragraph offering advice or a warning. Share one or two examples aloud (voluntarily) and ask the following questions if there's time: • What was the most important consequence you would want others to be aware of? • Did anything surprise you in today's lesson? • Do you feel more confident in recognising and avoiding risky situations?

<table>
<tr>
<td>Assessment Ideas</td>
<td colspan="3">Starter Activity
Use pupil responses in the brief scenario-based activity to gauge prior understanding of the legal and social consequences of substance misuse. Listen for misconceptions around the severity or nature of consequences (e.g. assuming minor legal repercussions or overlooking long-term social impact). Use this to identify key areas to revisit or reinforce during the lesson.
Main Activity
Observe group discussions as pupils analyse each case study. Look for their ability to identify and explain the specific legal and social consequences presented. Assess how well they justify their responses using evidence from the scenarios and their ability to explore alternative outcomes. Use their summaries and class contributions to evaluate critical thinking, empathy and their understanding of cause and effect in real-life contexts.
Plenary
During the final class discussion, assess which case studies pupils found most impactful and why. Look for thoughtful reasoning, use of appropriate language and the ability to articulate links between decisions, behaviours and consequences. This reflection provides insight into pupils' developing awareness of the broader implications of substance misuse.</td>
</tr>
<tr>
<td rowspan="2">Signposting and Support</td>
<td rowspan="2"><u>Website Support</u>
Talk to Frank: Offers confidential advice, facts and support about drugs and the law. Particularly useful for clarifying legal consequences.
www.talktofrank.com
Phone: 0300 123 6600
Childline: Free, confidential support for young people.
www.childline.org.uk
Phone: 0800 1111
Citizens Advice: Offers clear, age-appropriate guidance on criminal records, the law and rights. Useful for exploring long-term social consequences.
www.citizensadvice.org.uk</td>
<td>Cross-Topic Links</td>
<td>Law, psychology, sociology, citizenship</td>
</tr>
<tr>
<td>Teacher Confidence Tips</td>
<td>Familiarise yourself on current laws and social policies related to substance abuse before the lesson. Being well-informed will help you confidently address pupils' questions and correct misconceptions.</td>
</tr>
</table>

	<u>**School Support**</u> **School counsellor or pastoral lead**: Encourage pupils to speak confidentially to trusted staff if they have concerns about themselves, family or friends. **Local youth support services or police liaison officers**: Where possible, signpost or invite professionals to speak on the real-world legal implications and support pathways.		Establish clear ground rules for respectful discussion, especially since legal and social consequences can be sensitive topics. This helps you manage difficult conversations with confidence. Drawing on relevant case studies or news stories can make the lesson more relatable and engaging. It also gives you concrete reference points to guide discussions.

5 KS5: Lesson Plans

KS5 Lesson 1

<table>
<tr><td rowspan="2">Lesson Title</td><td rowspan="2">Alcohol and Other Drugs</td><td>Key Stage</td><td>5</td></tr>
<tr><td>Lesson Length</td><td>50 minutes</td></tr>
<tr><td colspan="4">Lesson Objectives</td></tr>
<tr><td colspan="4">• Explain the physical, mental, social and legal effects of alcohol and other commonly used substances.
• Analyse how societal attitudes and personal beliefs influence perceptions of substance use.
• Evaluate the consequences of substance use on individuals and wider communities.
• Apply critical thinking to challenge common myths and stereotypes about drugs and alcohol.</td></tr>
<tr><td>Resources Needed</td><td>• Statement cards or slides
• Interactive whiteboard (if presenting slides)
• Access to reliable websites like Talk to Frank, Drinkaware
• Case file worksheets/ templates
• Devices with internet access (optional)</td><td>Key Vocabulary</td><td>Alcohol, substance, legal and illegal drugs, mental health, stigma, harm reduction, peer pressure, coping strategies, social consequences, physical health effects, risk</td></tr>
<tr><td>Creating Learner Agreement</td><td colspan="3">Begin the lesson by establishing a positive and respectful classroom environment through the creation of a learner agreement. This sets clear expectations for behaviour, participation and respect, helping all pupils feel safe and engaged.

Briefly explain to pupils that the learner agreement is a set of shared rules everyone agrees to follow during the lesson (and ideally, throughout the series). Emphasise that this helps create a respectful space where everyone can learn and express their views safely.</td></tr>
</table>

DOI: 10.4324/9781003608998-5

	Invite pupils to contribute their ideas about what makes a good learning environment. Prompt with questions like • What behaviours help us learn best? • How can we respect each other's opinions? • What should we do if someone is disruptive? As pupils suggest behaviours, write these on the board or a visible flipchart. Typical points might include • Listen when others are speaking. • Respect different opinions. • Stay on task and participate. • Use appropriate language. • Keep phones away unless instructed (if applicable). Refer to this agreement at the start of every lesson to reinforce expectations.
Starter Activity (10 minutes)	Display the following three statements on the board or printed handout: **A.** Using alcohol responsibly means you're in control. **B.** Society's attitude towards legal drugs is more harmful than the drugs themselves. **C.** People who misuse drugs are responsible for their choices, regardless of their background. Ask pupils to choose one statement they feel strongly about, whether they agree, disagree or are unsure and write a short personal response: • Do you agree or disagree? Why? • What assumptions does this statement make? • Can you think of any real-world examples that support or challenge it? In groups of 3–4, pupils share their responses. Encourage respectful debate: • Where do their views align or differ? • What experiences or values shape these views? • Can they challenge each other's thinking constructively? Bring the class back together and invite a few pupils to share insights from their group: • Which statement sparked the most disagreement? • What made the conversation interesting or surprising? • How do these views influence the way we talk about alcohol and drugs in society?

<table>
<tr>
<td>Main Activity</td>
<td>
Divide the class into 4–5 small groups, ideally with 3–5 pupils each. Assign or allow each group to choose one substance from the following list:
• Alcohol.
• Cannabis.
• MDMA (ecstasy).
• Cocaine.
• Nitrous Oxide (laughing gas).

If pupils have studied some of these in KS4, encourage them to dig deeper by looking at more nuanced or updated angles, such as
• Shifting legal frameworks (e.g. changes in cannabis classification).
• Links with social media, celebrity use or online misinformation.
• Latest statistics or harm-reduction data.
• High-profile cases or real-life scenarios involving the substance.

Provide each group with a case file worksheet (KS5 Lesson 1 Resource 1), which prompts them to examine their assigned substance through these key lenses:
• Physical health effects (short- and long-term).
• Mental health impacts (e.g. anxiety, depression, psychosis).
• Social consequences (e.g. friendships, family, work, reputation).
• Legal status and implications (possession, supply, sentencing).
• Cultural/media representation or recent debates (optional).

Groups can conduct research using school-approved devices or printouts.

Encourage pupils to consider both risks and realities, e.g. not just the legal penalties, but also how certain laws might disproportionately affect certain groups, or how media narratives can shape public perceptions.

Each group delivers a 2-minute summary of their findings, focusing on insightful takeaways rather than listing facts. Encourage them to clearly explain the following:
• One surprising or lesser-known fact.
• A key takeaway for their peers.
• A question or ethical dilemma that arose during research.

After each presentation, invite the class to ask 1–2 short questions, encouraging respectful challenge and deeper thinking. Use this as an opportunity to clarify misconceptions and highlight connections between substances.

This activity supports collaborative learning, public speaking, critical thinking, and empathy, which are all key elements of a robust KS5 PSHE curriculum.
</td>
</tr>
</table>

<table>
<tr><td>Plenary
(10 minutes)</td><td>Ask each pupil to complete the following two prompts silently on a sticky note, piece of paper, or in their books:
• One insight I'm taking away from today's lesson is . . .
• One question I still have about alcohol or other drugs is . . .

Encourage pupils to think critically and personally. Their insight might relate to
• A myth they've reconsidered.
• A fact that surprised them.
• A social impact they hadn't considered.
• A shift in how they view choices or responsibilities.

Their question might relate to
• Policy (e.g. Why is alcohol legal if it causes so much harm?).
• Identity (e.g. why do some people feel more pressure than others to use drugs?).
• Consequences (e.g. what support is actually available for people struggling with misuse?).

Invite a few volunteers to read either their insight or question aloud. Alternatively, do a quick 'Pass the Paper' where pupils swap them randomly and read one anonymously.

Finish by summarising the key theme of the lesson:

Today we moved beyond just learning about what substances do. We've begun asking why people use them, how society treats them and what the real consequences are. These aren't just legal or health issues. They're human, social and emotional too. Your questions will help shape our future lessons.

These questions from KS5 Lesson 1 can be
• Used at the start of future lessons as springboards.
• Turned into 'Your Questions Answered' slides.
• Addressed in mini-discussions or extension tasks during the lesson.</td></tr>
<tr><td>Assessment
Ideas</td><td>Starter Activity
Use pupil responses during the 'Challenging Perspectives' discussion to assess their ability to express and justify personal views about substance use. Listen for how confidently they draw on prior knowledge from KS4 and whether they can consider different viewpoints with maturity.

Main Activity
Observe group interactions during the 'Substance Case Files' investigation to assess how well pupils can identify, explain and analyse the physical, mental, social and legal impacts of substance use. Use open-ended questions to prompt deeper thinking and evaluate how pupils handle complex issues such as stigma, legality and societal attitudes in their presentations.</td></tr>
</table>

<table>
<tr><td></td><td colspan="3">Plenary
Review pupils' written reflections to assess their depth of understanding and ability to reflect critically. Look for insights that show meaningful engagement with the topic and questions that reveal curiosity, ethical thinking or misconceptions that may need addressing in future lessons.</td></tr>
<tr><td rowspan="2">Signposting and Support</td><td rowspan="2"><u>Website Support</u>
Talk to Frank: Offers confidential advice, facts and support about drugs and the law. Particularly useful for clarifying legal consequences.
www.talktofrank.com
Phone: 0300 123 6600
Drinkaware: A trusted source for alcohol facts, health risks and tips for making safer choices. Includes tools like unit calculators and real-life advice.
www.drinkaware.co.uk
YoungMinds: Mental health charity for young people. Includes support for those experiencing anxiety, low mood or substance-related worries.
www.youngminds.org.uk
The Mix: Support for under-25s covering drugs, mental health, relationships, legal rights and more. Offers a free helpline, forums and live chat.
www.themix.org.uk</td><td>Cross-Topic Links</td><td>Science/biology, physical health, mental health, citizenship, English</td></tr>
<tr><td>Teacher Confidence Tips</td><td>Set and remind pupils of respectful listening and no judgement, so everyone feels safe to share ideas or questions without fear.
Acknowledge what pupils already know from KS4 and earlier lessons to validate their experience and build on existing understanding.</td></tr>
</table>

	School Support **School counsellor or pastoral lead**: Offer confidential support for pupils concerned about their own or others' substance use. **Local youth offending team (YOT)**: Can be invited to speak or offer referrals when exploring legal consequences in more detail with KS5 pupils.		

KS5 Lesson 2

Lesson Title	The Science of Addiction	**Key Stage**	4
		Lesson Length	50 minutes
Lesson Objectives			
• Describe the key scientific factors involved in addiction, including brain chemistry, dependency and tolerance. • Explain the difference between physical and psychological addiction, and how both can develop. • Compare different models of addiction (biological, psychological and biopsychosocial) and explore how they help us understand individual experiences. • Reflect on how this knowledge connects to wider issues such as mental health, coping strategies and decision-making.			
Resources Needed	• Printed case studies • Addiction model summary handouts • Pens and paper or exercise books • Printed exit question slips interactive whiteboard	**Key Vocabulary**	Addiction, dependence, withdrawal, dopamine, brain reward system, physical addiction, psychological addiction, biological model, psychological model, biopsychosocial model, relapse, craving, triggers, genetic predisposition, environment, coping mechanisms, stigma, recovery

Starter Activity (10 minutes)	Review the learner agreement as a class. Present 6–8 statements related to addiction science. Pupils work in pairs or small groups to decide if each is a myth or fact or whether they are unsure, and briefly explain their reasoning. Here are some statements you could use: • Addiction is just a lack of willpower. • Addiction changes the structure and chemistry of the brain. • Only illegal drugs cause addiction. • Genetics play no role in addiction. • Withdrawal symptoms are purely psychological. • Social environment has no impact on addiction. After discussion, reveal answers and clarify misconceptions with short explanations.
Main Activity (30 minutes)	This activity helps pupils explore the complexity of addiction by applying different theoretical models to real-life case scenarios. By examining how each model interprets the causes and treatment of addiction, pupils can better understand the multifaceted nature of substance use and how this shapes public perception and intervention approaches. Begin by briefly introducing the three main models of addiction. Use simple, relatable language: • **Biological/disease model**: Sees addiction as a chronic brain disease influenced by genetics or brain chemistry. • **Psychological model**: Focuses on thoughts, behaviours and learned experiences, e.g. addiction as a coping strategy or habit. • **Biopsychosocial model**: A more holistic model combining biological, psychological and social factors. Distribute summary handouts outlining the core ideas, strengths and criticisms of each model. You can display key points on the board or use visual aids to support understanding. Clarify that these models are frameworks, not absolute truths. They help us understand addiction from different lenses. Divide pupils into small groups (3–4 pupils per group). Assign each group the following: • One case study (**KS5 Lesson 2 Resource 1**) illustrating a real or realistic story of someone experiencing addiction. • One model summary sheet (ensure variety across groups so all three models are represented in the class).

	Ask each group to • Read and discuss the case study carefully. • Identify how their assigned model would explain the person's behaviour and experiences (e.g. What caused this addiction?/What keeps it going?). • Consider whether their model highlights any **treatment implications** – e.g. would this model suggest therapy, medication, lifestyle change or social support? • Discuss the strengths and limitations of applying this model to the case. What does it explain well? What does it miss or overlook?
	Encourage groups to take notes on a mini whiteboard or A3 paper for their presentation. Offer discussion prompts or model-specific scaffolding questions for groups needing extra support. Each group gives a concise presentation (up to 4 minutes) outlining • A short summary of their case study. • How their assigned model explains the addiction. • Strengths and limitations of the model in this context. Encourage groups to explain in their own words rather than reading directly from the handouts. After each group presents, invite the rest of the class to ask questions, give feedback or offer alternative interpretations (e.g. How might another model explain this differently?). Highlight that addiction is complex and often rooted in a combination of brain chemistry, trauma, environment and personal coping strategies. Reinforce the idea that no single model fully explains every experience of addiction. If time allows and to consolidate learning, ask pupils to respond individually in writing to the following questions: • Which model do you personally find most convincing or helpful? Why? • How might your understanding of addiction models affect how you view people who struggle with substance use? • What does this suggest about how we should approach treatment and support? This personal reflection encourages critical thinking and empathy while reinforcing lesson content. This main activity builds pupils' analytical skills, encourages open-mindedness and helps them grasp the importance of using multiple perspectives when tackling complex health and social issues like addiction.

<table>
<tr>
<td>Plenary
(10 minutes)</td>
<td colspan="3">Ask pupils to respond to the following prompt:
'Based on what you've learned today, how should society approach addiction and why is it important to understand the science behind it?'
Encourage them to refer to
• At least one addiction model (e.g. biological, psychological, biopsychosocial).
• Something surprising or new they learned from the lesson.
• How this knowledge might change the way they view people who are addicted.</td>
</tr>
<tr>
<td>Assessment Ideas</td>
<td colspan="3">Starter Activity
Use pupil responses in the 'Myth or Fact' discussion to gauge prior understanding and identify misconceptions about addiction. Listen carefully to their reasoning to assess their current grasp of scientific concepts such as willpower, brain changes and the role of genetics and environment.
Main Activity
Observe group collaboration and how well pupils apply the addiction models to their case studies. Look for evidence of critical thinking, balanced analysis and the ability to explain scientific factors clearly. Use their presentations to assess how confidently and accurately they can compare biological, psychological and biopsychosocial perspectives.
Plenary
Review pupils' written reflections to assess their depth of understanding and ability to apply learning to real-world thinking. Look for use of key terminology, reference to addiction models and evidence of a shift toward empathy and informed perspectives.</td>
</tr>
<tr>
<td rowspan="2">Signposting and Support</td>
<td rowspan="2"><u>Website Support</u>
Talk to Frank: Offers confidential advice, facts and support about drugs and the law. Particularly useful for clarifying legal consequences.
www.talktofrank.com
Phone: 0300 123 6600
Kooth: A free, anonymous online counselling and emotional well-being platform for 11–25 year olds. Includes self-help content, forums and live chat with qualified professionals.
www.kooth.com</td>
<td>Cross-Topic Links</td>
<td>Science/biology, mental health, citizenship, English, psychology</td>
</tr>
<tr>
<td>Teacher Confidence Tips</td>
<td>This lesson is about exploring concepts, not delivering a science lecture. Focus on helping pupils understand how addiction works You're guiding critical thinking, not teaching A-level biology.</td>
</tr>
</table>

	YoungMinds: Mental health charity for young people. Includes support for those experiencing anxiety, low mood or substance-related worries. www.youngminds.org.uk **The Mix**: Support for under-25s covering drugs, mental health, relationships, legal rights and more. Offers a free helpline, forums and live chat. www.themix.org.uk **School Support** **School counsellor or pastoral lead**: Offer confidential support for pupils concerned about their own or others' substance use. **Designated safeguarding lead (DSL)**: If something shared in this lesson is worrying, the DSL is there to help and support pupils' confidentially.		Use the case studies and model summaries to anchor discussions. You only need to cover the basic mechanisms: brain reward pathways (like dopamine), physical and psychological dependence, and how environment and genetics interact. Addiction affects people from all walks of life. Set a respectful, non-judgemental tone early on. This encourages open conversation and helps if pupils share personal thoughts or experiences.

KS5 Lesson 3

<table>
<tr><td>Lesson Title</td><td rowspan="2">Drug Use Rates and Global Society</td><td>Key Stage</td><td>4</td></tr>
<tr><td></td><td>Lesson Length</td><td>50 minutes</td></tr>
<tr><td colspan="4">Lesson Objectives</td></tr>
<tr><td colspan="4">• Analyse global data on drug use rates and identify patterns across different countries and regions.
• Explain how cultural, social, economic and legal factors influence drug use and policy variations worldwide.
• Compare and evaluate different countries' approaches to drug policy, considering their social and health impacts.
• Develop critical thinking and data literacy skills by interpreting news articles and statistics.</td></tr>
<tr><td>Resources Needed</td><td>• News article extracts from diverse countries (use of devices, if possible)
• Data summaries on drug use rates and policies
• Pens and paper or exercise books
• Printed or digital world map (optional)
• Interactive whiteboard</td><td>Key Vocabulary</td><td>Drug use rates, decriminalisation, legalisation, policy, cultural norms, stigma, addiction, rehabilitation, relapse, global health, imprisonment, public health, death penalty</td></tr>
</table>

<table>
<tr><td>Starter Activity</td><td>
Review the learner agreement as a class.

Display a blank world map (printed or projected).

Ask pupils, individually or in pairs, to write down or discuss what they think about drug use in different parts of the world. For example,
• Which countries might have higher or lower drug use rates?
• How might government policies differ (e.g. prohibition, decriminalisation, harm reduction)?
• What cultural or societal factors could influence drug use and attitudes?

Invite some pupils to share their ideas and place brief notes or symbols on the map to highlight key points.

Use this as a springboard to introduce the lesson topic, exploring real data and global social contexts.
</td></tr>
<tr><td>Main Activity</td><td>
This activity helps pupils understand how drug use and policy vary across the world. It encourages critical thinking about how political, legal, cultural and economic factors shape substance-related outcomes. Pupils will analyse real-world data, compare international case studies and consider what ‘effective’ drug policy might look like.

Introduce the activity with context. You might say,

Every country handles drug policy differently. Some focus on punishment, others on treatment or education. Today, you’ll explore how these different approaches affect societies, including drug use rates, public health, crime and well-being.

Explain that pupils will work in pairs, with each pair analysing one country’s policy and outcomes.

Each pair should then receive the following:
• A short article extract or summary describing one country’s approach to drug policy. Use age-appropriate sources that reflect a range of viewpoints.
• A simple data summary (charts, bullet points or infographic) showing recent drug use statistics, overdose rates or trends in that country.

Suggested countries and themes:
• Portugal: Decriminalisation model and public health outcomes.
• United States of America: Opioid crisis and addiction treatment challenges.
• Netherlands: Tolerance of cannabis and regulated sale.
• Singapore: Zero-tolerance laws and harsh penalties.
• Brazil: Drug-related violence and social inequality.
</td></tr>
</table>

	You may wish to pre-group pupils strategically to support differentiation or language needs. In pairs, pupils read their article and study the data. Provide clear discussion prompts on the board or in handout form (**KS5 Lesson 3 Resource 1**). Ask them to make notes on the following: • What is the country's approach to drug use and policy? • What impact has this had on the population or public health? • What social, cultural, legal or economic factors might explain the drug use rates? • What are the strengths and weaknesses of this country's approach? • How does this compare with what they know about drug policy in the United Kingdom or elsewhere? Circulate to support pairs. Encourage pupils to think beyond surface-level observations and ask clarifying or challenging questions. After discussion, each pupil writes a 150–200 word summary that includes the following: • A brief overview of their assigned country's current situation. • A critical evaluation of the policy's effectiveness. • One personal reflection or key takeaway (e.g. 'I was surprised by . . .' or 'This made me reconsider . . .'). You can use writing frames or sentence starters for support: • In [Country], the government's approach to drug use is . . . • One of the outcomes of this policy has been . . . • I believe this approach is effective/ineffective because . . . Pairs swap their written responses with another pair and read about a different country's approach. Encourage them to discuss • Similarities and differences. • What surprised or challenged them. • Which policy they found most compelling and why. This broadens their exposure beyond their own article and promotes critical comparisons. Invite a few pairs to share highlights from their country analysis. Then facilitate a guided class discussion using open-ended questions: • Which approach seemed most effective overall? Why? • Do harsher penalties reduce drug use or push it underground? • How do culture, law and social systems influence drug outcomes? • Should all countries adopt the same approach or tailor their own? Encourage pupils to explore complexity, challenge assumptions and reflect on harm reduction, public health and justice.

<table>
<tr><td></td><td colspan="3">This activity supports pupils in developing global awareness, evidence-based reasoning and ethical thinking which are all essential skills for informed citizenship and health literacy.</td></tr>
<tr><td>Plenary</td><td colspan="3">Ask pupils to spend 5–7 minutes writing a short response to this prompt:
Considering what we've learned today about drug use rates and policies around the world, how might your perspective on drug use and policy have changed? What is one thing you think governments or societies should do differently, and why?
• Invite a few pupils to share their thoughts if they feel comfortable.
• Reinforce the idea that drug use and policy are complex, interconnected issues requiring empathy, evidence and open-mindedness.</td></tr>
<tr><td>Assessment Ideas</td><td colspan="3">Starter Activity
Use pupil contributions to the world map discussion to gauge their initial understanding of global drug use perceptions and cultural influences.
Main Activity
Assess pairs' written analyses for their ability to interpret data, critically evaluate different countries' drug policies and make comparisons. Observe discussions to check for development in critical thinking, cultural awareness and empathy.
Plenary
Review pupils' written reflections to assess how well they can articulate changes in perspective, propose informed policy ideas, and demonstrate nuanced understanding of global drug issues.</td></tr>
<tr><td rowspan="2">Signposting and Support</td><td rowspan="2"><u>Website Support</u>
Talk to Frank: Reliable information about drugs, including global perspectives and local support.
www.talktofrank.com
Phone: 0300 123 6600
Kooth: Free, anonymous online counselling and emotional well-being support for young people
www.kooth.com</td><td>Cross-Topic Links</td><td>Geography, sociology, citizenship, law, physical health</td></tr>
<tr><td>Teacher Confidence Tips</td><td>Choose news articles that present a range of perspectives, including successes, challenges and controversies, to avoid bias and encourage critical thinking.</td></tr>
</table>

	YoungMinds: Mental health charity for young people. Includes support for those experiencing anxiety, low mood or substance-related worries. www.youngminds.org.uk **The Mix**: Support for under-25s covering drugs, mental health, relationships, legal rights and more. Offers a free helpline, forums and live chat. www.themix.org.uk **School Support** **School counsellor or pastoral lead**: Offer confidential support for pupils concerned about their own or others' substance use. **Designated safeguarding lead (DSL)**: If something shared in this lesson is worrying, the DSL is there to help and support pupils' confidentially.		Be prepared for personal disclosures; know your school's safeguarding procedures and have support signposting ready. Let pupils lead discussions but step in to guide and challenge thinking with probing questions or to keep conversations on track.

KS5 Lesson 4

Lesson Title	The Impact of Substance Abuse on Mental Health	**Key Stage**	5
		Lesson Length	50 minutes
Lesson Objectives			
• Define what is meant by *dual diagnosis* and explain the link between substance abuse and mental health. • Explore how substance use can affect mood, behaviour and long-term mental well-being. • Analyse real-life scenarios to identify the complex relationship between substance use and psychological distress. • Suggest appropriate support or interventions for someone facing co-occurring substance and mental health challenges.			
Resources Needed	• Access to YouTube • Printed case studies support/ intervention handout • Paper or exercise books for written reflections • Whiteboard and markers • Optional slides for discussion prompts • Printed or digital exit slips	**Key Vocabulary**	Dual diagnosis, substance abuse, mental health, depression, anxiety, self-medication, addiction, trauma, intervention, recovery, co-occurring disorders, emotional well-being, psychological distress, relapse, support services, diagnosis, treatment, coping mechanisms, stigma, vulnerability

<table>
<tr><td>Starter Activity (10 minutes)</td><td>Review the learner agreement as a class.
Display this statement and question to the class:
'Substance abuse and mental health issues often feed into each other in complex ways. Can you think of some reasons why this might happen?'
In pairs, pupils discuss the question for a few minutes.
Encourage them to consider different perspectives (biological, psychological, social).
Ask them to think about why some people might turn to substances when struggling with mental health and how substance use might worsen mental health problems.
After discussion, pupils write a short reflection (3–4 sentences):
Summarise their main thoughts or any new insights from the discussion.
Here are some ideas for sentence starters for the reflections:
• One reason substance abuse and mental health are connected is because . . .
• A challenge for people struggling with both substance use and mental health might be . . .
• I think substance use can affect mental health by . . .
• It's important to understand that mental health problems can sometimes lead to substance use because . . .
• After our discussion, I realise that the relationship between substance abuse and mental health is . . .
Invite a few pairs to share key points with the class to kick off a wider conversation.</td></tr>
<tr><td>Main Activity</td><td>Start by showing this short explainer video:
Co-occurring Disorders: Mental Health and Substance Use
https://www.youtube.com/watch?v=CZajlQUWdFc
Before pressing play, introduce the video in accessible language:
Today we're looking at how mental health challenges and substance use can happen at the same time. This is called a co-occurring or dual diagnosis. This video will help explain what that means, how these conditions can interact and why it makes recovery more complex.
Encourage pupils to jot down any key points or terminology they hear during the video that stands out or feels important.</td></tr>
</table>

	Group Case Study Task (25–30 minutes) Split the class into small groups of 3–4 pupils. Give each group a fictional case study (**KS5 Lesson 4 Resource 1**) featuring a young person experiencing both mental health difficulties and problematic substance use. Choose relatable, age-appropriate scenarios, such as • A university student using alcohol to manage anxiety, leading to depression. • A young adult with bipolar disorder whose drug use worsens their mood swings. • A person recovering from childhood trauma misusing prescription painkillers. • A teenager caught in a cycle of addiction and relapse, affecting their self-worth. Alongside each case, provide a 1-page info sheet (**KS5 Lesson 4 Resource 2**) summarising common intervention options (e.g. cognitive behavioural therapy, peer support groups, GP involvement, harm reduction strategies, helplines). Ask groups to work through the following questions: • What mental health challenges are evident? • How might the substance use be connected to these issues? • What difficulties might this person face trying to get help? • Which types of support might actually work for them, and why? Encourage groups to refer to the support sheet and discuss with empathy, curiosity and without judgement. Circulate during the task to support discussions, challenge assumptions, and guide groups to consider both emotional and practical barriers to recovery. Once discussion ends, each pupil writes a 200–250 word analysis of their group's case study. This written piece should include the following: • A brief summary of the individual's situation. • An explanation of how mental health and substance use interact in the scenario. • At least two realistic support strategies or interventions that could help the person move toward recovery. Offer sentence starters for pupils who need scaffolding, such as • The main mental health issue in this case is . . . • Substance use makes this worse by . . . • A helpful support strategy might be . . .

<table>
<tr><td></td><td>Invite volunteers to read their analysis aloud or display a few anonymised examples. Use this as a springboard for a short whole-class discussion. Prompt pupils to think about
• What patterns did we notice across the different case studies?
• Why might it be hard to get help when mental health and substance use overlap?
• How can we make sure our support for others is kind, realistic and informed?
This activity supports critical thinking, empathy and deeper understanding of a complex but vital topic in a safe and accessible way.</td></tr>
<tr><td>Plenary (10 minutes)</td><td>Ask pupils to write a brief exit reflection (3–4 sentences) answering this prompt:
In your own words, explain why understanding the link between substance abuse and mental health (dual diagnosis) is important when supporting someone struggling with these issues.
Invite a few volunteers to share their reflections aloud to reinforce key ideas and end the lesson on a thoughtful note.</td></tr>
<tr><td>Assessment Ideas</td><td>Starter Activity
Use pupil reflections from the initial pair discussion to gauge their prior understanding of how substance abuse and mental health interact.
Main Activity
Observe group discussions and review written case study analyses to assess pupils' ability to identify dual diagnosis, explain the interplay between substance use and mental health, and suggest appropriate support or interventions.
Plenary
Evaluate pupils' exit reflections to check their understanding of why recognising the link between substance abuse and mental health is crucial for effective support.</td></tr>
</table>

<table>
<tr>
<td rowspan="2">Signposting and Support</td>
<td rowspan="2"><u>Website Support</u>
Talk to Frank: Reliable information about drugs, including global perspectives and local support.
www.talktofrank.com
Phone: 0300 123 6600
Kooth: Free, safe, anonymous online counselling and emotional well-being platform for young people.
www.kooth.com
YoungMinds: Mental health charity for young people. Includes information on anxiety, depression, trauma and where to get help.
www.youngminds.org.uk
The Mix: Support for under-25s covering topics like drugs, mental health, relationships and self-care.
www.themix.org.uk
<u>School Support</u>
School counsellor or pastoral lead: Offer confidential support for pupils who may be worried about their own or someone else's substance use or mental health.
Designated safeguarding lead (DSL): If something shared in this lesson is worrying, the DSL is there to help and support pupils' confidentially.</td>
<td>Cross-Topic Links</td>
<td>Mental health,
science/biology, sociology, citizenship,
psychology</td>
</tr>
<tr>
<td>Teacher Confidence Tips</td>
<td>This topic may be close to home for some pupils. Create a safe, respectful space and remind pupils they can step out or speak privately if they need support.
If you're not a specialist, focus on helping pupils understand how mental health and substance use can interact, rather than using complex clinical terms.
Frame the case studies and reflections in a way that helps pupils understand people's experiences, not judge them.</td>
</tr>
</table>

KS5 Lesson 5

Lesson Title	Debate: Drug Testing at Festivals Saves Lives	**Key Stage**	5
		Lesson Length	50 minutes
Lesson Objectives			
• Critically examine the arguments for and against drug testing at music festivals. • Use evidence to support a reasoned viewpoint on a complex, real-world issue. • Understand the principles of harm reduction and how they relate to personal and public safety. • Engage respectfully in structured debate, listening and responding to alternative perspectives.			
Resources Needed	• Evidence packs or curated news articles presenting pro and con arguments • Access to YouTube • Printed debate preparation sheets • Opinion continuum template (**KS5 Lesson 5 Resource 1**) • Mini whiteboard • Pens and paper • Interactive whiteboard (optional)	**Key Vocabulary**	Drug testing, harm reduction, legalisation, festival safety, public health, ethics, personal freedom, stigma, peer pressure, overdose, informed consent

Starter Activity (10 minutes)	Review the learner agreement as a class. Set up the continuum using templates as follows: Define one side of the room as **'Strongly Agree'** and the opposite as **'Strongly Disagree.'** The middle is **'Unsure/Neutral.'** **Read this prompt to the class:** 'I believe that providing free, anonymous drug-testing kits at music festivals saves lives.' Pupils quietly place themselves along the line according to their view. Encourage genuine placement. This is about their instinctive reaction before the debate. Once in position, each pupil pairs with someone next to them. They explain briefly to each other why they chose that spot, telling each other any personal or prior knowledge. Invite 2–3 volunteers from different points on the line to share their reasoning. Note any immediate concerns or assumptions on the board (e.g. 'reduces harm,' 'encourages use,' 'legal implications'). Also, make a note of pupils that did not understand the statement.
Main Activity	**Debate: Should Drug Testing Be Available at Festivals?** Begin by playing the video: *Will Drug Testing Tents at Music Festivals Improve Safety?* https://youtu.be/WvVDWcN-7fg?si=BDTMJUirEmbHmpUo This short video introduces pupils to the concept of on-site drug testing at festivals and sets the tone for a critical exploration of harm reduction, legality and public health. Next, split the class into two or four small groups, depending on size. Each group will take on a position: • **Pro** (in favour of drug testing). • **Con** (against drug testing). You may have multiple groups on the same side to encourage varied arguments. **Preparation Materials** Provide each group with an evidence pack or selection of short, accessible news articles. These should include the following: • Case studies of UK-based drug testing services (e.g. The Loop). • Arguments around harm reduction versus normalising drug use. • Legal perspectives (e.g. drug classification laws, festival liabilities). • Statistics on festival-related drug deaths or hospitalisations. • Examples of international models (e.g. Portugal, the Netherlands).

Research and Planning

Give pupils structured headings to organise their research and talking points:

- **Public health**: Does drug testing reduce risk and improve safety?
- **Legal/ethical**: Does testing create liability? Could it be seen as condoning use?
- **Youth safety**: What about young people who feel pressure to experiment?
- **Festival culture**: Is this a realistic and necessary intervention?
- **Personal freedom**: Where should personal responsibility begin and end?

Encourage pupils to assign speaking roles (e.g. introduction, evidence, rebuttal, conclusion) and prepare the following:

- A clear opening statement that outlines their group's position.
- 3–4 key arguments, supported with evidence.
- Anticipated counterarguments and thoughtful responses.
- A strong closing statement to summarise their case.

Pupils can use a debate planning sheet to organise their arguments (**KS5 Lesson 5 Resource 1**).

Debate Format

Each group presents their case. You can use a formal debate format (timed statements, rebuttals) or a more conversational approach, depending on the dynamic of your group. Set clear ground rules for respectful discussion and ensure each pupil has a chance to speak.

Circulate during preparation time to guide groups, clarify terminology and encourage critical engagement. Offer sentence starters or vocabulary prompts for pupils struggling with confidence.

If time allows, return to the original debate prompt (e.g. 'Should drug testing be offered at festivals?') and invite pupils to write or discuss whether their perspective has changed. Encourage them to consider

- What argument was most persuasive and why?
- Did anything surprise them?
- How does this relate to real-world decision-making for young people?

This activity is designed to build empathy and critical thinking and articulate reasoning. These are all crucial skills for navigating complex, real-life issues around substance use and personal safety.

<table>
<tr><td>Plenary (10 minutes)</td><td colspan="3">Ask pupils to individually respond to the following prompt in their exercise books or on a printed exit slip:

After taking part in the debate and hearing different perspectives, what is your current view on drug testing at festivals? Has your opinion changed or stayed the same? Explain why, using at least one argument or piece of evidence that influenced your thinking.

Encourage them to
• Acknowledge whether their view shifted or remained firm.
• Reference something said during the debate or found in the evidence pack.
• Comment on the strength or weakness of arguments they heard.

Ask a few pupils to voluntarily share whether their view evolved or not, and why. This helps highlight critical thinking and reinforces the value of evidence-informed opinions.</td></tr>
<tr><td>Assessment Ideas</td><td colspan="3">Starter Activity
Use pupils' positioning on the opinion continuum and their paired discussions to assess prior knowledge, ethical reasoning and initial attitudes toward harm reduction strategies.

Main Activity
Observe how pupils structure their arguments and engage in the debate. Look for clarity of thought, use of evidence, ability to respond to counterpoints and respectful discussion skills. Use questioning during or after the debate to prompt deeper evaluation of key issues.

Plenary
Assess how pupils' understanding has evolved by comparing their initial opinion with a written exit slip, reflection or group summary. Look for thoughtful evaluation of the debate and any shift in perspective based on evidence.</td></tr>
<tr><td>Signposting and Support</td><td><u>Website Support</u>
Talk to Frank: Honest and accessible information about drugs, including harm reduction strategies and festival safety advice.

www.talktofrank.com

Childline

Free, confidential

Phone: 0300 123 6600</td><td>Cross-Topic Links</td><td>Personal safety, politics, citizenship, media studies,

mental health,

first aid,

law, English</td></tr>
</table>

	The Loop: A UK-based harm reduction charity offering drug safety testing and education at festivals and clubs. www.wearetheloop.org **YoungMinds**: Support for young people's mental health, with advice on managing anxiety around festivals, peer pressure and well-being. www.youngminds.org.uk **The Mix**: Support for under-25s covering topics like drugs, mental health, relationships and self-care. www.themix.org.uk **<u>School Support</u>** **School counsellor or pastoral lead**: Available to support pupils who may be reflecting on their own or peers' substance use, especially in social settings like festivals or parties. **Designated safeguarding lead (DSL)**: Point of contact if any disclosures or concerns arise during or after the debate, particularly around drug use, peer pressure, or unsafe environments.	**Teacher Confidence Tips**	Remind pupils that the purpose of the debate is to explore different perspectives. Thoughtful reasoning is just as valuable as a 'winning' argument. Encourage pupils to back up their ideas with evidence and reassure them that changing your mind based on new information is a strength, not a weakness. Reassure pupils that debating is a skill, and every opportunity builds confidence, whether they speak today or just listen and learn.

KS5 Lesson 6

<table>
<tr><td>Lesson Title</td><td>Handling Parties, Nightclubs and Festivals</td><td>Key Stage</td><td>5</td></tr>
<tr><td></td><td></td><td>Lesson Length</td><td>50 minutes</td></tr>
<tr><td colspan="4">Lesson Objectives</td></tr>
<tr><td colspan="4">• Identify common risks associated with parties, festivals and nightclubs, including substance use, peer pressure and safety concerns.
• Apply harm reduction strategies to realistic scenarios, with a focus on staying safe and supporting others.
• Evaluate the impact of individual decisions in high-risk social environments and reflect on personal boundaries.
• Plan practical steps to prepare for and manage real-life events confidently and responsibly.</td></tr>
<tr><td>Resources Needed</td><td>• Printed or digital safety planning templates
• Case study scenario sheets
• Whiteboard or flipchart
• Post-it notes</td><td>Key Vocabulary</td><td>Proactive safety, peer pressure, personal safety, consent, emergency response, boundaries, intoxication, risk assessment, nightlife, festival culture, alertness, decision-making, support networks, spiking, safe exit strategies, buddy system, bystander intervention, prevention</td></tr>
<tr><td>Starter Activity (10 minutes)</td><td colspan="3">Review the learner agreement as a class.

Display or hand out a few realistic but anonymised scenarios (KS5 Lesson 6 Resource 1). Ask pupils to discuss
• What would you do in this situation?
• What factors might influence your decision?
• What would a safe or confident response look like?

Example Scenarios:
• You're at a festival and your friend has taken something but now feels unwell. They beg you not to tell anyone.
• You're offered a drink by someone you've just met in a club, and you didn't see it being poured.
• Your mates want to stay at an after-party, but you're tired, uncomfortable and don't know the people there.
• A friend is pressuring you to take something 'just to try it once, everyone's doing it.'</td></tr>
</table>

	Encourage pupils to be honest. There's no shame or 'right' answer but prompt discussion on • Personal safety. • Peer pressure. • Knowing when and how to walk away. • Trusting instincts. • Strategies for handling tricky social dynamics.
Main Activity (40 minutes)	Now it's time to get pupils thinking practically, collaboratively and with empathy. Organise the class into pairs or small groups of 3–4. Explain that their challenge is to design a realistic party safety plan for a night out. This could be a music festival, a house party or a night at a club. The focus here is not to tell pupils what *not* to do, but to give them space to reflect, plan and problem-solve, using real-world thinking that helps them make safer choices and look out for others. Distribute the Party Safety Plan Template (**KS5 Lesson 6 Resource 2**) and share a few example scenarios or event cards to help get them started. Alternatively, let them pick their own setting. Some pupils may prefer to plan for a chilled gathering at a friend's house, while others might imagine a lively festival. Encourage them to choose something that feels relevant or realistic to them. Make it clear that this is about proactive safety and support, not preaching or punishment. The aim is to think ahead, anticipate risk and create strategies that feel authentic and achievable. Ask each group to address the following key areas in their plan: • **Pre-event prep**: Who's going? How will they stay in touch? Are phones charged? What's the transport plan? What happens if someone gets separated from the group? Do they have an agreed backup plan or meeting point? • **During the event**: How will they handle peer pressure or unexpected offers of substances? What strategies can they use to keep one another safe (e.g. buddy systems, designated non-drinker, checking in regularly)? What signs might tell them that someone in the group isn't coping? • **If things go wrong**: How would they recognise that someone might need help (e.g. signs of overdose, panic attack or distress)? Who would they contact? Security, a safe zone, parents, emergency services? What would be the immediate steps they could take to keep someone safe? • **Post-event**: What does 'checking in' look like the next day? Are there conversations that need to be had? Can they reflect on what went well or what they'd change next time?

	Encourage depth and detail. Surface-level plans like 'we'll be careful' or 'we won't drink too much' aren't enough. Circulate the room, ask open-ended questions, and gently challenge vague responses. Use prompts like • What does that look like in practice? • How would you feel if that happened to a friend? • What's your plan if someone says they're fine but clearly isn't? This task should feel grounded in empathy as much as logistics. Pupils should imagine real conversations, real decisions and the real emotions that might come into play. Invite them to consider how their group might respectfully disagree and how they'd navigate that in the moment. **Wrap-up options:** Once groups complete their plans, you can either invite them to present their ideas to the class (great for practising communication and persuasion) or run a silent gallery walk, where plans are displayed and pupils circulate, reading each other's work and leaving written feedback or sticky-note questions. This activity offers an opportunity for critical thinking, peer learning and meaningful reflection, all through a lens of safety, autonomy and care.
Plenary (10 minutes)	Ask pupils to reflect quietly on everything they've discussed and planned during the lesson. Then, use this prompt: 'What is one thing you'll do differently, or think about more carefully, the next time you're at a party, festival or night out?' They should write their answer anonymously and honestly. It could be a personal boundary, a safety step or a way they'll support others. You can either • Collect responses in a box or stick them to a board/wall (anonymously). • Invite a few volunteers to share out loud. • Use mini whiteboards for a quick, non-verbal show of learning.
Assessment Ideas	**Starter Activity** Use pupil responses during the initial class discussion to gauge existing attitudes and assumptions about nightlife, peer dynamics and personal safety. **Main Activity** Observe how pupils engage in group discussions. Assess their ability to identify risks; apply harm reduction strategies; and offer practical, empathetic ideas. Look for evidence of collaborative thinking, real-world awareness and maturity in their planning.

<table>
<tr><td></td><td colspan="3">Plenary
Review pupil reflections to assess personal insight, responsibility and how well they internalised the lesson's message. Responses can inform your understanding of individual pupil readiness and future PSHE priorities.</td></tr>
<tr><td rowspan="2">Signposting and Support</td><td rowspan="2"><u>Website Support</u>
Talk to Frank: Honest and accessible information about drugs, including harm reduction strategies and festival safety advice.
www.talktofrank.com
Phone: 0300 123 6600
Drinkaware: Practical tools and information about alcohol, including safety tips for going out, how to spot danger signs and where to get help.
www.drinkaware.co.uk
The Mix: Support for under-25s covering topics like drugs, relationships, sexual health and staying safe on nights out.
www.themix.org.uk
<u>School Support</u>
School counsellor or pastoral lead: Offer confidential support for pupils concerned about risky situations, peer pressure or decisions they've made around parties and festivals.
Designated safeguarding lead (DSL): Important point of contact if a pupil discloses harm, unsafe experiences, or concerns about someone else's welfare following a night out.</td><td>Cross-Topic Links</td><td>Personal safety, citizenship,
media studies,
mental health,
first aid, English</td></tr>
<tr><td>Teacher Confidence Tips</td><td>KS5 pupils respond best to honesty and practical advice. Focus on empowering them to make safer decisions, not scaring them.
Remind pupils that the goal is to reduce risk and look out for each other, regardless of the choices people make. This creates a non-judgemental learning space.
Reference real-life examples (festivals, headlines, apps like 'Find My Friends') to anchor learning in familiar, relevant territory.</td></tr>
</table>

6 KS3: Tutor Time Plans

KS3 Tutor Time 1

<table>
<tr><td rowspan="2">Session Title</td><td rowspan="2">What Counts as Harmful?</td><td>Key Stage</td><td>3</td></tr>
<tr><td rowspan="2">Linked Lesson Plan</td><td rowspan="2">KS3 Lesson 1
Introduction to Harmful Substances</td></tr>
<tr><td>Session Length</td><td>15–20 minutes</td></tr>
<tr><td colspan="4">Intended Learning Focus</td></tr>
<tr><td colspan="4">To explore the range of substances considered harmful and reflect on why they are dangerous, even if they are legal or commonly used.
This tutor time session aims to help pupils explore and identify various substances that are considered harmful. Pupils will reflect on the difference between legality and safety and begin thinking critically about the consequences of using or misusing substances, including those that are socially accepted or prescribed.</td></tr>
<tr><td>Resources Needed</td><td colspan="3">• Quiz statements (printed or on slides/whiteboard)
• Whiteboards/Post-its and pens</td></tr>
<tr><td>Warm-Up Question</td><td colspan="3">Use the following question as a discussion prompt:
'Is something still harmful if it's legal or sold in shops?'
Ask pupils to consider common substances like alcohol, cigarettes, caffeine and energy drinks. Invite responses using think-pair-share or open class discussion.
Examples for discussion
• Alcohol is legal for adults, but drinking too much can damage your liver and affect mental health.
• Vaping products are sold in shops, but can harm your lungs, especially in young people.
• Some energy drinks contain high levels of caffeine and sugar that can cause sleep problems and heart issues.
Tutor talking point
Not everything that's legal is safe. Being informed helps to make responsible choices.</td></tr>
</table>

DOI: 10.4324/9781003608998-6

<table>
<tr><td>Recap Activity</td><td>Use this quiz to challenge misconceptions and check baseline understanding. Pupils can answer using thumbs up/down, whiteboards, or by moving to designated corners (True/False).

Quiz statements and explanations

1. All harmful substances are illegal. (False)

Many harmful substances are legal but can be dangerous if misused (e.g. alcohol, solvents or even some over-the-counter medications).

2. Alcohol can be harmful to the body. (True)

Excessive alcohol use can cause liver damage and mental health issues and increase the risk of accidents.

3. Prescription drugs are always safe. (False)

They are only safe when taken as prescribed by a doctor. Misuse, even with good intentions, can be very dangerous.

Follow-up questions to extend understanding
• Can you name a legal substance that can be harmful?
• Why do you think some harmful substances are still sold?</td></tr>
<tr><td>Character and Values Reflection</td><td>Discussion prompt
'Why does responsibility matter when it comes to substances?'

Possible pupil responses
• Because I'm in control of what I put in my body.
• Someone might get hurt if they don't understand what they're taking.
• If I know something's harmful, I should help my friends avoid it too.

Tutor talking points
• Responsibility means making choices that are safe for you and those around you.
• If someone offers you a substance, being responsible means knowing the risks and making your own decision.
• Think about how your choices could affect your health, school life, family and friendships.</td></tr>
<tr><td>Exit Question</td><td>'What's one harmful substance you've heard about that surprised you?'
• Prompt them to consider something they assumed was harmless or didn't know much about before (e.g. codeine, nitrous oxide, caffeine).

This encourages personal reflection and critical thinking while highlighting lesser-known risks.</td></tr>
</table>

Extension Activity	**Creative challenge** Pupils can create a slogan warning people about a lesser-known harmful substance.	**Differentiation and Tips**	Support younger or less confident pupils with sentence starters during discussion. Offer example slogans or visuals to prompt ideas. For EAL pupils, provide key terms (e.g. harmful, prescription, substance) with definitions or visuals.

KS3 Tutor Time 2

Session Title	Drugs: Medicine or Misuse?	**Key Stage**	3
		Linked Lesson Plan	KS3 Lesson 2 Medicinal versus Recreational Drugs
Session Length	15–20 minutes		
Intended Learning Focus			
To help pupils understand the difference between medicines that help us when used properly and substances that can cause harm when misused. The session encourages personal reflection, builds awareness of responsible behaviour and promotes informed choices about drug use.			
Resources Needed	• Printed list or slide with substances for the sorting activity • Post-it notes or whiteboards for quick reflection • Paper, pens and coloured pencils for the extension posters		
Warm-Up Question	Use the following question as a discussion prompt: 'Have you ever had to take medicine? How did it help you?' This question can be used as a think-pair-share discussion or a short class conversation. If more structure is needed, ask pupils to write one sentence about a time they took medicine and what the result was. **Tutor talking points** • Most pupils will have experience with medicine like antibiotics, painkillers or inhalers. • Emphasise that medicine is designed to help the body recover or manage conditions.		

	Examples might include • I had an ear infection, and antibiotics helped me feel better. • I took allergy tablets so I could focus in class. • My asthma inhaler helps me breathe when my asthma is playing up. Ensure pupils understand that medicines, when used as intended, are helpful and often essential, but they can also be dangerous if misused.
Recap Activity	**Activity Title: 'Medicinal or Recreational?'** Give pupils a list of substances (either read out loud, shown on a slide or on a handout) and ask them to identify whether each one is • **Medicinal** (used to treat illness). • **Recreational** (used for pleasure, not health, often illegal or harmful). **Examples to include** • **Paracetamol**: Medicinal. • **Cannabis**: Both (explain that it can be misused). • **Cough syrup**: Medicinal. • **Cocaine**: Recreational. • **Codeine**: Both (explain that it can be misused). • **Inhaler**: Medicinal. • **Alcohol**: Recreational. • **Antibiotics**: Medicinal. **Follow-up discussion** Ask pupils the following questions: • Why might some substances appear in both categories? • What could happen if a medicine is used when it's not needed or not prescribed? **Teaching point** Some substances (like codeine or certain allergy meds) are helpful when used as prescribed but dangerous if overused or used recreationally.
Character and Values Reflection	**Discussion Prompt** 'How does responsibility apply to using medicine?' **Pupil responses might include** • You shouldn't take more than you're told to. • If you feel better, you still have to finish the course of antibiotics. • I would tell an adult if someone offered me pills that weren't mine.

<table>
<tr><td></td><td colspan="3">Talking points to guide discussion
• Being responsible means following the instructions from a doctor or pharmacist.
• Being responsible means never sharing medicine with someone it wasn't prescribed for.
• Responsibility includes knowing when not to take something, even if others around you are.
• Responsibility is about making choices that protect your health and support the well-being of others. Misusing medicine can cause harm to your body, your judgement and even your future.</td></tr>
<tr><td>Exit Question</td><td colspan="3">'What's one rule you think is important for safe medicine use?'
Pupils can answer via
• Post-it notes for the learning wall.
• Verbal feedback.
• Individual written responses on mini whiteboards.
Examples of good answers
• Always read the label.
• Only take what's prescribed to you.
• Ask a trusted adult if you're unsure.
The purpose of this activity is to help reinforce the idea that safe medicine use isn't just about what we take, it's about how, when and why we take it.</td></tr>
<tr><td>Extension Activity</td><td>Creative challenge
Create a mini-poster entitled 'Safe Medicine Habits'
Pupils should choose one or two important safety rules. They should decorate the poster with visuals like a medicine bottle, showing safe versus unsafe behaviour. You could select winning posters to hang on the wall of the tutor group room</td><td>Differentiation and Tips</td><td>Pair EAL or SEND pupils with peers for group discussion.
Provide word banks with key vocabulary, e.g. dosage, prescription, overdose, side effects.
Offer templates for the poster if pupils need more structure.</td></tr>
</table>

KS3 Tutor Time 3

<table>
<tr><td>Session Title</td><td>Energy Drinks: Fuel or False Boost?</td><td>Key Stage</td><td>3</td></tr>
<tr><td>Session Length</td><td>15–20 minutes</td><td>Linked Lesson Plan</td><td>KS3 Lesson 3
Over-Consumption of Energy Drinks</td></tr>
<tr><td colspan="4">Intended Learning Focus</td></tr>
<tr><td colspan="4">To help pupils understand what's in energy drinks, the possible negative effects of over-consumption and to reflect on healthier ways to boost energy and stay focused. This session promotes informed decision-making and builds awareness around common but misunderstood habits.</td></tr>
<tr><td>Resources Needed</td><td colspan="3">• True or false quiz (printed or shown on screen)
• Paper and coloured pens/pencils for posters
• Post-it notes or whiteboards for reflection</td></tr>
<tr><td>Warm-Up Question</td><td colspan="3">Use the following question as a discussion prompt:
'Why do you think people drink energy drinks?'
Possible discussion strategies:
• Think-pair-share or group discussion.
• Ask pupils to call out reasons or write their ideas on Post-its or whiteboards.
Common answers may include
• To feel more awake.
• They think it gives them energy for sports or gaming.
• Because they taste good.
• To stay up late or revise.
Tutor talking points
• These reasons are understandable, especially for teenagers under pressure.
• However, many people don't fully understand what energy drinks contain or how they affect the body.
Transition line
Let's take a look at what's really inside these drinks and why too much can be a problem.</td></tr>
</table>

<table>
<tr><td>Recap Activity</td><td>Activity Title: 'What's in an Energy Drink?'
• Thumbs up/down or A/B/C cards for quick responses.
Quiz questions (with answers and short facts)
1. How much sugar can be in one large energy drink (500ml)?
A) 1 teaspoon
B) 5 teaspoons
C) 13 teaspoons (Correct)
That's over double the recommended daily amount for teenagers.
2. Which ingredient in energy drinks acts as a stimulant?
A) Vitamin C
B) Caffeine (Correct)
C) Calcium
Some drinks contain more caffeine than three cups of coffee.
3. What is a possible emotional side effect of too much caffeine?
A) Calmness
B) Anxiety (Correct)
C) Drowsiness
Too much caffeine can lead to anxiety, restlessness or irritability.
4. Which of these is a healthier way to increase energy levels?
A) Sleeping well (Correct)
B) Drinking energy drinks
C) Skipping breakfast
When you have finished the quiz, ask pupils this question:
'Were you surprised by any of those answers?'
Briefly highlight the short- and long-term effects: jitteriness, poor sleep, sugar crashes and increased heart rate.</td></tr>
<tr><td>Character and Values Reflection</td><td>Discussion prompt
'Why is self-control helpful when making food and drink choices?'
Pupil responses might include
• You need to think about how it'll make you feel later.
• If I'm tired, maybe I should sleep instead of drinking caffeine.
• Self-control helps you stay focused on what's good for you.</td></tr>
</table>

<table>
<tr><td></td><td colspan="3">Ideas to explore in discussion
• Self-control means thinking before acting, especially when a choice feels tempting but may not be good for you.
• It's easy to follow trends (e.g. grabbing an energy drink before school or during revision), but good choices often come from awareness and planning.
• Choosing water or food over energy drinks can protect your mood, sleep and long-term health.</td></tr>
<tr><td>Exit Question</td><td colspan="3">'What's a healthier way to boost your energy?'
Options for pupil response could be
• Written on whiteboards or Post-its.
• Shared aloud with the group.
• Written in a reflection journal or tutor folder.
Expected ideas might include
• Drinking water.
• Going outside for fresh air.
• Having a balanced snack.
• Getting more sleep.
• Exercising to wake up my body.
This question encourages pupils to make a personal connection and consider practical strategies they can use.</td></tr>
<tr><td>Extension Activity</td><td>Creative challenge
Design an advert for a healthy alternative to energy drinks.
Pupils can choose a healthier substitute, e.g. fruit smoothie, water, banana, nuts or simply sleep/rest. They can also create a catchy slogan, fact, or image to promote it. Remind them their alternative should highlight what it does for your energy and focus, without the crash or risk.</td><td>Differentiation and Tips</td><td>Pair EAL or SEND pupils with peers for group discussion.
Provide word banks with key vocabulary, e.g. dosage, prescription, overdose, side effects.
Offer templates for the poster if pupils need more structure.</td></tr>
</table>

KS3 Tutor Time 4

<table>
<tr><td>Session Title</td><td>Vaping: What's the Real Story?</td><td>Key Stage</td><td>3</td></tr>
<tr><td>Session Length</td><td>15–20 minutes</td><td>Linked Lesson Plan</td><td>KS3 Lesson 4
The Risks of Vaping and E-Cigarettes</td></tr>
<tr><td colspan="4">Intended Learning Focus</td></tr>
<tr><td colspan="4">To challenge common myths about vaping and to encourage responsible decision-making and peer awareness.</td></tr>
<tr><td>Resources Needed</td><td colspan="3">• Printed quiz questions or slides
• Post-its or whiteboards
• Paper and art supplies for the extension challenge (optional)</td></tr>
<tr><td>Warm-Up Question</td><td colspan="3">Use the following question as a discussion prompt:
'Why might someone start vaping even if they know it's risky?'
Use a think-pair-share activity. Ask pupils to think individually, discuss with a partner and then share ideas with the class.
Possible responses may include
• They think it's safer than smoking.
• Their friends are doing it.
• They're curious or want to try it.
• They like the flavours.
• They believe it helps with stress or boredom.
Tutor talking points
• Many young people start vaping even if they've heard that it might be harmful.
• There are lots of mixed messages online and in social media.
• It's important to understand what fact is and what myth is. We will explore that today.</td></tr>
<tr><td>Recap Activity</td><td colspan="3">Activity Title: 'What's True About Vaping?'
Deliver a short true/false quiz to challenge common misconceptions and provide quick facts.
Quiz questions
1. Vaping is completely safe because it doesn't contain tobacco. (False)
While vaping doesn't involve burning tobacco, it often contains nicotine and other harmful chemicals.</td></tr>
</table>

<table>
<tr><td></td><td colspan="3">2. You can get addicted to vaping. (True)
Most vapes contain nicotine, which is highly addictive, especially for young people.
3. Flavoured vapes are harmless because they taste like sweets. (False)
Flavours may make vaping feel less serious, but they still contain substances that affect lungs and brain development.
4. Vaping can affect concentration, sleep and mental health. (True)
Nicotine can disrupt sleep, increase anxiety and reduce focus.
5. Most pupils your age are vaping regularly. (False)
Many pupils overestimate how common vaping is. The majority of teenagers don't vape.</td></tr>
<tr><td>Character and Values Reflection</td><td colspan="3">Discussion prompt
'Why is it brave to say no?'
Pupil responses may include
• It's hard to be different, but I know what's best for me.
• It's brave to stand up for yourself.
• It's easier to follow the crowd. Saying no shows independence.
Discussion ideas
• Saying no when others are pressuring you takes confidence and strength.
• It's brave to do what's right for you, even if others disagree.
• Peer pressure is real, but self-respect and long-term thinking are more important.</td></tr>
<tr><td>Exit Question</td><td colspan="3">'What's one fact about vaping you'd share with a friend?'
Pupils can write on a Post-it note or a mini whiteboard.
This exit question encourages pupils to become peer mentors and build the confidence to challenge misinformation.</td></tr>
<tr><td>Extension Activity</td><td>Creative challenge
Get pupils to design a poster that busts that uses facts, visuals and a strong message about vaping. They should include a catchy slogan or attention-grabbing design.</td><td>Differentiation and Tips</td><td>Provide key vocabulary for EAL/SEND pupils (e.g. nicotine, addiction, peer pressure).
Offer sentence starters for reflection (e.g. 'One thing I learned today is . . .').
Allow pair or group work for the creative task to support confidence.</td></tr>
</table>

KS3 Tutor Time 5

<table>
<tr><td>Session Title</td><td>Peer Pressure</td><td>Key Stage</td><td>3</td></tr>
<tr><td>Session Length</td><td>15–20 minutes</td><td>Linked Lesson Plan</td><td>KS3 Lesson 5
Understanding Peer Pressure</td></tr>
<tr><td colspan="4">Intended Learning Focus</td></tr>
<tr><td colspan="4">To reflect on how peers can influence decision-making and to develop strategies for staying true to personal values.</td></tr>
<tr><td>Resources Needed</td><td colspan="3">• Printed scenario cards or list for reading aloud
• Post-it notes and pens
• Display board or wall space for extension task (optional)</td></tr>
<tr><td>Warm-Up Question</td><td colspan="3">Use the following question as a discussion prompt:
'What does peer pressure feel like?'
Ask pupils to consider their thoughts silently for 30 seconds, then discuss with a partner or small group. Afterward, invite a few responses to be shared aloud.
Pupil responses may include
• It feels like everyone expects you to do something.
• Like you'll be left out if you don't join in.
• Like you'll get judged or laughed at.
• It can feel exciting but scary at the same time.
Tutor talking points
• Peer pressure can be both positive and negative.
• It's natural to want to fit in, but it's also important to make decisions that match your values.
• Today's session is about recognising those moments and learning how to respond.</td></tr>
<tr><td>Recap Activity</td><td colspan="3">Activity Title: 'What Kind of Pressure?'
Read out a series of short scenarios. Pupils decide whether each one is positive peer pressure or negative peer pressure.
Delivery Options
• Pupils vote using thumbs up/down.
• Use mini whiteboards to display answers.
• Discuss each scenario as a class or in small groups.</td></tr>
</table>

	Sample Scenarios • **Your friend encourages you to revise with them after school.** Positive: Encouraging good habits. • **A group dares you to try vaping so you don't seem 'boring.'** Negative: Encouraging risky behaviour. • **Your classmate invites you to join a new sports club.** Positive: Supportive influence. • **Someone mocks you for not drinking at a party.** Negative: Pressure through embarrassment. • **Your friend reminds you not to cheat on homework.** Positive: Encouraging honesty. **Discussion prompt** • What makes the difference between helpful and harmful pressure? • Can you think of a time when you've seen or felt either kind?
Character and Values Reflection	**Discussion prompt** 'How can you stay true to your values?' **Suggested pupil responses could include** • I remind myself what I care about. • I talk to someone I trust before making big decisions. • I walk away from situations that don't feel right. • I ask myself, 'Would I regret this later?' **Reflection talking points** • Your values are your beliefs about what's right and important. • Knowing your values makes it easier to say no when something doesn't feel right. • It's not always easy to speak up, but practising how to respond can help.
Exit Question	**'What's one way to stand up for yourself in a tricky situation?'** Get pupils to write down their ideas on paper or Post-it notes. Share answers in pairs or as a whole class. **Examples of pupil responses** • Say no politely but firmly. • Change the subject or walk away. • Tell a trusted adult if something feels wrong. • Support someone else who's being pressured. This exit question should leave pupils with a specific, practical strategy they can use in real-life situations.

Extension Activity	**Creative challenge** Post-it Wall: Phrases to Say When You Want to Say No Pupils each write one or two short phrases on Post-it notes that could help them say no in a kind but confident way. Stick the Post-its on a class 'Power to Say No' wall or display board. **Examples of phrases** • No thanks, that's not for me. • I'd rather not. • I'm not into that. • Let's do something else. • I'm good, thanks.	**Differentiation and Tips**	Provide sentence starters for reflections and responses (e.g. 'One way I can stand up for myself is . . .'). Offer quiet pair discussion for pupils less confident speaking aloud. Use visuals or keywords to support EAL/SEND access.

KS3 Tutor Time 6

Session Title	Addicted to Likes?	**Key Stage**	3
Session Length	15–20 minutes	**Linked Lesson Plan**	KS3 Lesson 6 Debate: Is Social Media as Harmful as Drugs and Alcohol for Mental Health?
Intended Learning Focus			
To explore how social media can affect our emotions, mental well-being and ability to focus and to reflect on how to build a healthier digital life.			
Resources Needed	• Statement cards or quiz slides • Post-it notes or whiteboards • Display materials for pledge poster		

Warm-Up Question	**Use the following question as a discussion prompt:** 'How does it feel when someone likes your post?' Begin with individual reflection. Ask pupils to consider how they feel when they receive attention online, such as likes, comments or views. Then invite small groups or pairs to share and discuss their thoughts. **Pupil responses may include** • It makes me feel good about myself. • It's exciting! I want to check my phone again. • It depends who liked it. • I feel disappointed if I don't get many. • It gives me a confidence boost. **Tutor talking points** • Social media can create positive feelings, but it can also make us feel anxious, distracted or left out. • Today's session is about recognising how it affects us and how to stay in control of how we use it.
Recap Activity	Read out a series of behaviours. Pupils must decide whether each is helpful or unhelpful for their mental well-being. You can use thumbs up/down, whiteboards or group discussion to vote. **Statements to sort** • **I check my likes every five minutes, even during lessons.** Unhelpful: Distracting and can increase anxiety. • **I only post things that make my life look perfect.** Unhelpful: Can create pressure and unrealistic standards. • **I take regular breaks from my phone**. Helpful: Allows time for rest, focus and real-life connection. • **I use social media to keep in touch with friends in other places.** Helpful: Maintains relationships in a positive way. • **I feel sad or jealous when I see others' posts.** Unhelpful: Common, but something we can work on recognising and managing. • **I follow accounts that make me feel positive and inspired.** Helpful: Uplifting content can boost mood. **Discussion prompt** 'Which one of these do you relate to most, and why?'

<table>
<tr><td>Character and Values Reflection</td><td colspan="3">Discussion prompt
'How can you look after your mental wellbeing online?'
Pupil responses may include
• I put my phone away before bed.
• I've turned off notifications.
• I unfollowed accounts that made me feel bad.
• I take a break when I feel overwhelmed.
Reflection talking points
• Be mindful of how you feel before and after scrolling.
• Set time limits or screen breaks.
• Follow people who inspire you, not stress you out.
• Don't compare your real life to someone else's highlight reel.</td></tr>
<tr><td>Exit Question</td><td colspan="3">'What's one way you could use social media more positively?'
Ways to share
• Pupils write on paper, mini whiteboards or Post-it notes.
• Share a few aloud with the class.
• Add responses to a classroom display or journal.
Possible responses
• Use it to share kind messages.
• Follow pages that teach me something.
• Only post when I want to, not just for likes.
• Limit screen time so I can sleep better.
This question will encourage ownership of social media habits and a positive outlook.</td></tr>
<tr><td>Extension Activity</td><td>Creative challenge
Create a Class 'Digital Balance' Pledge
As a class, create a shared list of positive digital behaviours to support mental well-being.
Each pupil contributes one idea for balance, kindness or safety online.
Combine the ideas into a pledge and display in the tutor room.</td><td>Differentiation and Tips</td><td>Provide vocabulary support (e.g. well-being, comparison, notification).
Offer visual prompts or sentence starters, e.g. 'One positive thing I can do online is . . .'
Allow verbal responses for pupils who prefer to speak rather than write.</td></tr>
</table>

7 KS4: Tutor Time Plans

KS4 Tutor Time 1

<table>
<tr><td rowspan="2">Session Title</td><td rowspan="2">Substances and Their Impact: What's the Real Cost?</td><td>Key Stage</td><td>3</td></tr>
<tr><td rowspan="2">Linked Lesson Plan</td><td rowspan="2">KS4 Lesson 1 Understanding the Effects of Common Substances</td></tr>
<tr><td>Session Length</td><td>15–20 minutes</td></tr>
<tr><td colspan="4">Intended Learning Focus</td></tr>
<tr><td colspan="4">To revisit and reflect on the physical, emotional and social effects of commonly used substances such as alcohol, tobacco, cannabis and others. Pupils will explore the gap between perception and reality and consider how knowledge shapes healthier choices.</td></tr>
<tr><td>Resources Needed</td><td colspan="3">• Quiz statements (printed or on slides/whiteboard)
• Whiteboards/Post-its and pens</td></tr>
<tr><td>Warm-Up Question</td><td colspan="3">Use the following question as a discussion prompt:
'Why do some people still use substances even when they know the risks?'

Ask pupils to silently reflect for 30 seconds, then share their thoughts in pairs or small groups. Gather a few insights to share with the whole class.

Pupil responses may include
• They want to fit in with friends.
• They don't think anything bad will happen to them.
• They're curious or bored.
• They use it to relax or escape problems.
• They don't know the full risks.

Tutor talking points
• People's choices are influenced by many factors: social pressure, habits, misinformation or emotional challenges.
• Even if risks are known, they can seem distant or unlikely.
• That's why honest education and reflection are key.

Remind them that not all substances that are legal are safe. Being informed helps to make responsible choices.</td></tr>
</table>

DOI: 10.4324/9781003608998-7

Recap Activity	**Multiple-choice quiz (5–6 minutes)** Pupils answer individually using mini whiteboards or paper, or hands up. **Quiz questions** • **Which substance is most linked to long-term lung damage?** A. Alcohol B. Cannabis C. Tobacco (Correct) • **What's a short-term effect of cannabis use?** A. High blood pressure B. Impaired memory and coordination (Correct) C. Lung infection • **Can alcohol affect mental health?** A. Yes (Correct) B. No C. Only in large amounts • **True or False: All legal substances are safe.** False. Legal doesn't always mean harmless.
Character and Values Reflection	**Discussion prompt** 'Why does self-awareness matter when it comes to choices about health?' **Pupil reflection examples** • If I know I get stressed before exams, I can plan better coping strategies. • When I notice I'm feeling pressured, I can choose to walk away. • Being aware of how substances affect me or others helps me think more clearly. **Reflection talking points** • Self-awareness means recognising your triggers, habits, influences and values. • Being aware of why you're tempted by a choice makes it easier to step back and make a healthier decision. • It's about learning to pause and reflect, even when others might not.

Exit Question	**'What's one risk about a common substance that people should talk about more?'** Pupils write their answers on a slip of paper or Post-it and then share in pairs or choose a few to read aloud anonymously. **Possible responses** • How alcohol affects mental health. • Addiction can start with small habits. • Cannabis might seem harmless, but it can affect memory and focus. • Tobacco is still the biggest cause of preventable deaths. This question will promote a shift from general awareness to specific, actionable understanding, helping pupils become better equipped to make informed decisions.		
Extension Activity	**Creative challenge** In the centre of a page, write the name of a substance. Around it, draw **five ripple zones or branches** labelled • Physical health. • Mental health. • Relationships. • School/work life. • Future plans. Pupils then write or sketch **one consequence** for each area.	**Differentiation and Tips**	Allow pupils to choose between writing, drawing or discussing their ideas. Extend higher ability pupils by asking them to compare the risks of multiple substances or challenge common myths.

KS4 Tutor Time 2

Session Title	Influencers, Filters and Confidence	**Key Stage**	3
Session Length	15–20 minutes	**Linked Lesson Plan**	KS3 Lesson 2 Managing Peer/Media Influence and Self-Esteem
Intended Learning Focus			
To reflect on how social media and peer groups influence body image, self-worth and decision-making.			

Resources Needed	• Mini whiteboards and pens • Paper or card for the extension display
Warm-Up Question	**Use the following question as a discussion prompt:** 'Have you ever changed something about yourself based on what you saw online?' Ask pupils to think silently for 30 seconds, then share with a partner. Encourage a few volunteers to share with the whole group if comfortable. Validate all responses and guide toward the idea that online influence can be both subtle and powerful. Remind pupils that social media shows highlights – not reality. Many online images are filtered, staged or heavily edited.
Recap Activity	Read out or display each statement. Pupils decide whether each one reflects a **helpful** or **harmful** influence. **Statements (examples)** • Everyone drinks at parties. • Only perfect bodies get likes. • It's okay to say no to a trend. • You need to post constantly to stay popular. • Confidence means being yourself, not copying others. • I feel bad when my photo doesn't get likes. Pupils show thumbs up (helpful) or down (harmful). They then work in pairs to discuss and then provide feedback. **You could then ask** • Why do you think some harmful messages are so believable? • Which of these do you think young people see most often?
Character and Values Reflection	**Discussion Prompt:** 'How can self-respect protect you from negative influence?' Give a definition: *Self-respect means valuing yourself enough to make choices that protect your well-being.* Ask pupils to reflect on the following: • One way I can show self-respect online is . . . • A time I ignored pressure because I trusted myself was . . . **Pupil reflection examples** • Unfollowing toxic accounts. • Choosing not to join in with an unkind trend. • Wearing what they like, not just what's trending.

<table>
<tr><td>Exit Question</td><td colspan="3">'What's one influence you want to be more aware of this week?' Pupils jot their response on a Post-it note or journal card. Invite volunteers to share anonymously.</td></tr>
<tr><td>Extension Activity</td><td>Creative challenge Each pupil writes 1–2 positive, real things they like about themselves.
Encourage a mix of character strengths (e.g. kindness, humour, effort) and non-appearance-based traits.
Display responses on a 'Wall of Confidence' or classroom board.</td><td>Differentiation and Tips</td><td>Provide sentence starters.
Offer quiet pair or small group discussion for pupils less confident speaking aloud.
Use visuals or keyword prompts to support EAL/SEND access.
Challenge more confident pupils to explore how media influences work (e.g. algorithms, beauty standards, peer norms).</td></tr>
</table>

KS4 Tutor Time 3

<table>
<tr><td>Session Title</td><td>Coping or Escaping?</td><td>Key Stage</td><td>3</td></tr>
<tr><td>Session Length</td><td>15–20 minutes</td><td>Linked Lesson Plan</td><td>KS4 Lesson 3
Psychological Reasons for Drug Use and Healthy Coping Strategies</td></tr>
<tr><td colspan="4">Intended Learning Focus</td></tr>
<tr><td colspan="4">To explore the emotional reasons behind substance misuse and introduce healthier, more resilient ways of coping with stress and emotions.</td></tr>
<tr><td>Resources Needed</td><td colspan="3">• Printed or displayed matching activity cards (or list on board/slide)
• Sticky notes or small reflection cards
• Paper and pens for the self-care poster
• Optional: pre-made 'self-care menu' templates</td></tr>
</table>

<table>
<tr><td>Warm-Up Question</td><td>Use the following question as a discussion prompt:
'What are some reasons people might turn to substances to cope?'

Encourage pupils to brainstorm individually or in pairs. Accept a range of emotional and situational triggers: stress, anxiety, peer pressure, loneliness, boredom and trauma. Highlight that while some people believe substances help in the short term, they often worsen emotional well-being over time.

You may also want to ask
'What might someone be trying to escape by using substances?'</td></tr>
<tr><td>Recap Activity</td><td>Matching activity
Present pupils with pairs of behaviours. Ask them to match the unhealthy coping strategy with a healthier alternative.

You can do this verbally or on a mini whiteboard.

Examples
• Substance use ↔ Talking to someone you trust.
• Avoiding problems ↔ Making a realistic plan.
• Bottling up feelings ↔ Journaling or creative expression.
• Isolating ↔ Spending time with supportive people.
• Self-criticism ↔ Practising self-kindness.

Pupils match in pairs and share answers.

Follow-up discussion
• Why do you think some of the healthy strategies are harder to choose in the moment?
• Which healthy strategy do you think is most helpful in real life?</td></tr>
<tr><td>Character and Values Reflection</td><td>Discussion Prompt:
'What does resilience look like in tough times?'

Explain that resilience isn't about 'being strong' all the time. It's also about making choices that protect your well-being and help you bounce back.

Encourage responses like

• Knowing when to ask for help.

• Trying again after failing.

• Taking care of yourself even when life is stressful.

Ask pupils
'What's one small thing someone could do today that shows resilience?'</td></tr>
</table>

Exit Question	'What's one healthy coping strategy you could try this month?' Pupils write their answer on a Post-it note or reflection card. Share aloud if comfortable or drop anonymously into a reflection box. Revisit answers in a future session to follow up on progress.		
Extension Activity	**Creative challenge** Pupils design a mini-poster titled: 'My Self-Care Menu – 5 Ways I Cope Healthily.' Ideas they could include • Listening to music. • Talking to a friend or family member. • Going for a walk or exercising. • Drawing, journaling or writing. • Breathing exercises or mindfulness. • Doing something fun or relaxing. These could be displayed somewhere in the room to celebrate healthy choices.	**Differentiation and Tips**	**Adapt the matching task** with fewer or more simplified options for EAL/SEND pupils. **Challenge more able pupils** to explain *why* healthy strategies work or suggest how schools/families can encourage resilience.

KS4 Tutor Time 4

Session Title	Substances and Relationships: What's the Impact?	**Key Stage**	4
		Linked Lesson Plan	KS3 Lesson 4 Substances and Relationships
Session Length	15–20 minutes		
Intended Learning Focus			
To explore how substance use can affect relationships (friendships, family trust and romantic partnerships) and promote awareness of respectful, supportive connections.			

Resources Needed	• Printed or projected scenario cards for the healthy/harmful sort • Post-it notes or slips of paper for the takeaway and extension activities • Display board or wall space for 'What I Value in Relationships' (optional) • Pens, markers, decorative materials for display (optional)
Warm-Up Question	**Use the following question as a discussion prompt:** 'How can one person's behaviour affect their relationships with others?' Start with individual think time or silent journaling and then move into brief pair discussion. Take 2–3 whole-group responses and draw links to responsibility and emotional impact. **Tutor talking points** • Behaviour doesn't exist in a vacuum. Choices ripple outwards. • Trust, reliability and respect are affected by how we treat others (and ourselves).
Recap Activity	Present pupils with a set of short relationship scenarios. Ask them to identify whether the situation reflects a **healthy** or **harmful** relationship dynamic. **Here are a few examples:** • Your friend hides their drinking from their parents. • A partner pressures you to try something you're not comfortable with. • Someone opens up to you about wanting help to stop. • You lie to a parent to cover for a friend using substances. • A friend supports your decision not to drink at a party. Thumbs up/down or show of fingers (1 = healthy, 2 = harmful). Have a class discussion after each answer: 'Why do you think this is healthy or harmful?' The key concept to communicate here is that substance misuse can cause secrecy, loss of trust, manipulation and emotional stress, even for those not using the substance themselves.

<table>
<tr><td>Character and Values Reflection</td><td colspan="3">Discussion prompt
'What roles do honesty and trust play in strong relationships?'
Discussion prompts
• Why is trust so important in friendships and family life?
• What does it feel like when someone lies to protect their substance use?
• How can being honest, even when it's difficult, help relationships grow?
To find answers to these questions, pupils may use
1. Think-pair-share.
2. Sentence starters: 'A strong relationship means . . .' or 'Trust is important because . . .'</td></tr>
<tr><td>Exit Question</td><td colspan="3">'What's one way substance use could damage a relationship?'
Pupils write a response on a sticky note or index card.
Encourage honesty; this is a reflective, not judgemental, space.
Have the option to collect responses for anonymous display or to revisit next session.</td></tr>
<tr><td>Extension Activity</td><td>Creative challenge
Pupils write a word or phrase that represents what they value in a healthy relationship (e.g. trust, honesty, loyalty, space, kindness, forgiveness).
Use Post-it notes or decorate slips of paper.
Build a visual display that reinforces positive relationship values.</td><td>Differentiation and Tips</td><td>Provide sentence starters (e.g. 'One way substance use can harm a friendship is . . .', 'Trust matters because . . .').</td></tr>
</table>

KS4 Tutor Time 5

Session Title	Smoke-Free Future?	**Key Stage**	4
		Linked Lesson Plan	KS Lesson 5 Debate: Should There Be a Smoking Ban?
Session Length	15–20 minutes		
Intended Learning Focus			
To encourage pupils to engage in respectful discussion about public health versus personal freedom and to explore their own opinions on smoking bans.			
Resources Needed	Sentence starters to support discussion • 'I think smoking should/should not be banned because . . .' • 'One reason someone might disagree is . . .'		
Warm-Up Question	**Use the following question as a discussion prompt:** 'Should the government ban things that are bad for us, even if some people still want them?' Allow pupils to think-pair-share to allow quieter pupils time to gather thoughts. Ask for a few volunteers to share their opinions aloud. Encourage balanced thinking: personal freedom versus public health. You could also ask the following questions: • Are there any examples where this already happens? • What if banning something actually saves lives?		
Recap Activity	Pupils discuss one or more statements in pairs or small groups, giving a **Yes** or **No** response with reasons. Here are some debate prompts that you could use: 1. Should smoking be banned in public places like parks or outside schools? 2. Is vaping as dangerous as smoking traditional cigarettes? 3. Should tobacco be illegal for everyone under 25? 4. Would a full ban on smoking reduce health problems in the United Kingdom? Pupils can work in pairs to argue different sides. After they have debated, you could use a whole-class tally at the end: who agrees/disagrees and why? Ensure that pupils • Listen respectfully. • Use phrases like 'I understand your view, but I think . . .' or 'One reason I disagree is . . .'. • Focus on health impacts, social freedom and the role of government.		

<table>
<tr><td>Character and Values Reflection</td><td colspan="3">Discussion prompt
'Why does citizenship include thinking about what's fair for others, not just yourself?'
Discussion prompts
• Link to public health issues: second-hand smoke, younger people's exposure, NHS cost.
• Citizenship means balancing individual rights with community responsibility.
• Invite answers like
  • It's about protecting vulnerable people.
  • We all share public spaces, so fairness matters.
  • Sometimes we need rules to stop harm.
If time allows, get pupils to complete this sentence:
'Being a good citizen means . . .'</td></tr>
<tr><td>Exit Question</td><td colspan="3">'Where do you stand? Should smoking be banned completely? Why or why not?'
Pupils write down their position on a Post-it note or reflection card.
Encourage use of evidence or personal reasoning.</td></tr>
<tr><td>Extension Activity</td><td>Creative challenge
Pupils design a campaign slogan either for or against a full smoking ban.
Examples
• 'Breathe Easy: Ban Smoking for Good.'
• 'Freedom to Choose, Not to Lose.'
• 'Protect the Future: Smoke-Free Starts Now.'
• 'Adults Deserve the Right to Decide.'</td><td>Differentiation and Tips</td><td>Match more confident speakers with peers needing support.
Use sentence starters to support discussion:
• 'I think smoking should/ should not be banned because . . .'
• 'One reason someone might disagree is . . .'</td></tr>
</table>

KS4 Tutor Time 6

<table>
<tr><td rowspan="2">Session Title</td><td rowspan="2">Think Before You Risk It</td><td>Key Stage</td><td>3</td></tr>
<tr><td rowspan="2">Linked Lesson Plan</td><td rowspan="2">KS4 Lesson 6 Legal and Social Consequences of Substance Abuse</td></tr>
<tr><td>Session Length</td><td>15–20 minutes</td></tr>
<tr><td colspan="4">Intended Learning Focus</td></tr>
<tr><td colspan="4">To help pupils understand that risky behaviour involving substances can have long-term legal, social and personal consequences, beyond just immediate health effects.</td></tr>
<tr><td>Resources Needed</td><td colspan="3">• Statement cards or quiz slides
• Post-it notes or whiteboards
• Display materials for pledge poster</td></tr>
<tr><td>Warm-Up Question</td><td colspan="3">Use the following question as a discussion prompt:
'What kind of consequences can people face when they break laws about substances?'
Get pupils to silently reflect on this question, followed by pair-share.
Complete a class brainstorm on the board, grouped into legal, social and personal categories.
Pupils may mention
• Fines, arrest, criminal record.
• Loss of trust in relationships.
• Barriers to employment or travel.
• Damage to reputation or future opportunities.</td></tr>
<tr><td>Recap Activity</td><td colspan="3">Read each of these statements aloud (or display on board) and ask pupils to respond 'True' or 'False' with a show of hands, whiteboards or paired discussion.
Statements
• You can be prosecuted for having cannabis even if it's for personal use.
True: Cannabis is illegal for personal possession in the United Kingdom.
• Drug possession always leads to a criminal record.
False: Not always, but it can, depending on age, context and previous offences.
• Employers can refuse to hire you based on past substance offences.
True: Some jobs require DBS (disclosure and barring system) checks or have strict policies.</td></tr>
</table>

<table>
<tr><td></td><td colspan="3">• There's no social stigma with drug misuse anymore.
False: There is still judgement, fear and misunderstanding in many communities.
Invite short discussion after each question, clarifying any misconceptions and linking back to real-world consequences.</td></tr>
<tr><td>Character and Values Reflection</td><td colspan="3">Discussion prompt
'How does thinking ahead show maturity?'
Ask pupils to reflect quietly, then offer a few sentence starters:
• Thinking ahead helps me because . . .
• Being mature means considering . . .
Reflection talking points
• Maturity involves weighing the long-term impact of short-term decisions.
• Actions today (e.g. experimenting with substances) can affect education, work and relationships in future.</td></tr>
<tr><td>Exit Question</td><td colspan="3">'What's one consequence you hadn't really thought about before today?'
Pupils can write individual answers on Post-it notes or mini whiteboards. Examples might include travel restrictions, losing trust, not getting a job or hurting others.</td></tr>
<tr><td>Extension Activity</td><td>Creative challenge
Pupils create a simple flowchart that starts with one risky decision (e.g. accepting drugs at a party) and branches into multiple possible outcomes.
Encourage both short-term and long-term consequences:
• Legal trouble.
• Breaking trust with parents.
• Missing school.
• Social media reputation damage.
• Feeling regret.</td><td>Differentiation and Tips</td><td>Allow paired or group work for those who benefit from collaborative thinking.
Challenge higher-ability pupils to consider how consequences differ by age, class or background.</td></tr>
</table>

8 KS5: Tutor Time Plans

KS5 Tutor Time 1

<table>
<tr><td rowspan="2">Session Title</td><td rowspan="2">Alcohol and Other Drugs: Informed Decisions</td><td>Key Stage</td><td>5</td></tr>
<tr><td rowspan="2">Linked Lesson Plan</td><td rowspan="2">KS5 Lesson 1
Alcohol and Other Drugs</td></tr>
<tr><td>Session Length</td><td>15–20 minutes</td></tr>
<tr><td colspan="4">Intended Learning Focus</td></tr>
<tr><td colspan="4">To critically consider the short- and long-term effects of alcohol and drug use on both physical health and personal decision-making, especially in social contexts.</td></tr>
<tr><td>Resources Needed</td><td colspan="3">• Quiz statements (on slides, printed or read aloud)
• Mini-whiteboards for reflection
• Whiteboard or flip chart for the class brainstorm</td></tr>
<tr><td>Warm-Up Question</td><td colspan="3">Use the following question as a discussion prompt:
'Why do some risks seem acceptable in social situations?'
This should be a silent reflection followed by pair-share. Follow this with a group discussion with scribing key words on the board.
Here are some points you might want to mention if not raised:
• Peer pressure and social norms.
• Perception of invincibility or 'it won't happen to me.'
• Desire to fit in or avoid looking boring.
• Media influence and glamorisation of substances.</td></tr>
<tr><td>Recap Activity</td><td colspan="3">Read each of the following statements aloud. Pupils can vote true/false using mini whiteboards, thumbs up/down, or think-pair-share.
Statements
• Binge drinking can cause long-term brain damage.
True: It can damage brain development and memory, especially in young adults.
• Cannabis is legal for recreational use in the United Kingdom.
False: Cannabis is still illegal for recreational use in the United Kingdom.</td></tr>
</table>

DOI: 10.4324/9781003608998-8

	• **Mixing substances can multiply their effects.** True: Combining drugs (e.g. alcohol and depressants) can increase the risk of overdose and unpredictable reactions. Briefly explain the reasoning behind each answer to clarify misconceptions and reinforce learning.		
Character and Values Reflection	**Discussion prompt** 'How can self-control and responsibility guide your decisions when others are drinking or using drugs?' Here are some sentence starters they could use: • Being responsible means . . . • I can show self-control by . . . • One way to stay safe is . . . **Discussion prompts** • Delaying or declining participation. • Setting boundaries ahead of time. • Watching out for friends and being a role model. • Understanding your own limits and values.		
Exit Question	**'What's one way you can make a safer choice in a setting where alcohol or drugs are present?'** Pupils can produce written reflections on paper or mini whiteboards. **Here are a few examples that pupils might give:** • Agree a limit before going out. • Stay with friends I trust. • Offer to be the designated driver. • Know how to say no without pressure.		
Extension Activity	**Creative challenge** Ask pupils to design a short advice guide: '5 Ways to Stay Safe at Social Events,' either written or visual.	**Differentiation and Tips**	Quiet pair discussions for pupils who don't like sharing in front of a group. Visual support with keywords (e.g. risk, binge drinking, peer pressure) for EAL/SEND pupils.

KS5 Tutor Time 2

<table>
<tr><td rowspan="2">Session Title</td><td rowspan="2">Addiction: Choice or Chemistry?</td><td>Key Stage 5</td><td></td></tr>
<tr><td rowspan="2">Linked Lesson Plan</td><td rowspan="2">KS5 Lesson 2
The Science of Addiction</td></tr>
<tr><td>Session Length</td><td>15–20 minutes</td></tr>
<tr><td colspan="4">Intended Learning Focus</td></tr>
<tr><td colspan="4">To understand the neurological and psychological processes involved in addiction and challenge common misconceptions about choice, blame and brain response.</td></tr>
<tr><td>Resources Needed</td><td colspan="3">• Interactive whiteboard or display slide for sentence starters and keywords
• Pens, mini whiteboards or notebooks</td></tr>
<tr><td>Warm-Up Question</td><td colspan="3">Use the following question as a discussion prompt:
'Is addiction a choice or a brain condition?'

Get pupils to silently reflect followed by pair-share. Have a whole-group discussion to share ideas.

Points to explore
• Voluntary use can develop into involuntary behaviour.
• How repeated use changes the brain's reward system.
• The role of dopamine and habit loops.
• Social, emotional and environmental factors also play a part.

Ensure pupils understand that medicines, when used as intended, are helpful and often essential, but they can also be dangerous if misused.</td></tr>
<tr><td>Recap Activity</td><td colspan="3">Display or distribute the following sentence stems. Pupils complete them individually or in pairs.

Sentence Stems
1. Addiction is . . . (e.g. 'a brain condition that affects control over substance use or behaviour').
2. The brain reacts to substances by . . . (e.g. 'releasing chemicals like dopamine that make the user feel good – and want more').
3. One common myth about addiction is . . . (e.g. 'that it only happens to people with no willpower').

Pupils can write answers on Post-it notes or mini whiteboards. Share sentences as a whole class.</td></tr>
</table>

<table>
<tr><td>Character and Values Reflection</td><td colspan="3">Discussion prompt
'How does empathy shape how we respond to people struggling with addiction?'
If necessary, display a few sentence starters:
• Empathy helps me understand that . . .
• If someone I knew was struggling with addiction, I would . . .
• Judging someone doesn't help because . . .
Discussion themes
• Addiction isn't just a failure of willpower.
• Empathy leads to support, not shame.
• Supporting recovery requires understanding, not blame.</td></tr>
<tr><td>Exit Question</td><td colspan="3">'What's one thing you understand better about addiction after today?'
Get pupils to write a sentence or short phrase on a Post-it or index card.
Possible answers
• Addiction changes brain chemistry.
• People need support, not judgement.
• It can happen gradually and affect anyone.</td></tr>
<tr><td>Extension Activity</td><td>Creative challenge
'Is society too quick to judge or excuse addiction?'
Pupils discuss in pairs or small groups.
Encourage them to write down both sides of the argument.</td><td>Differentiation and Tips</td><td>Sentence starters for reflection activities
• Addiction happens because . . .
• Empathy helps because . . .
• I learned that . . .</td></tr>
</table>

KS5 Tutor Time 3

<table>
<tr><td>Session Title</td><td>Drugs Around the World: Culture, Context and Control</td><td>Key Stage</td><td>5</td></tr>
<tr><td>Session Length</td><td>15–20 minutes</td><td>Linked Lesson Plan</td><td>KS3 Lesson 3
Drug Use Rates and Global Society</td></tr>
<tr><td colspan="4">Intended Learning Focus</td></tr>
<tr><td colspan="4">To explore how drug use and laws differ between countries, why these approaches vary and what we can learn from them.</td></tr>
<tr><td>Resources Needed</td><td colspan="3">• Printed or digital map of the world (or Europe, if preferred)
• Matching cards or handout (Country ↔ Policy)
• Post-its or whiteboards for pupil responses
• Slide or print-out showing definitions of key policy types</td></tr>
<tr><td>Warm-Up Question</td><td colspan="3">Use the following question as a discussion prompt:
'Why do some countries have lower drug use despite more relaxed laws?'
Get pupils to think silently for 30 seconds and then share ideas in pairs or small groups. Invite a few comments to open the topic.
Key discussion points
• Cultural norms and education.
• Health-led approaches versus punishment.
• Public attitudes and stigma.</td></tr>
<tr><td>Recap Activity</td><td colspan="3">Get the pupils to match each country with its drug policy approach.
Country Policy Type
Portugal Decriminalisation
Sweden Zero tolerance
Netherlands Cannabis tolerated in cafés
USA Mixed – varies by state
Singapore Very strict, harsh penalties</td></tr>
</table>

<table>
<tr><td>Character and Values Reflection</td><td colspan="3">'How does open-mindedness help us understand different global approaches to drug use?'
Here are some suggestions for sentence starters:
• Being open-minded means . . .
• Different laws don't always mean better or worse, just . . .
• Understanding global policies helps me . . .
Get pupils to write this as an individual written reflection.</td></tr>
<tr><td>Exit Question</td><td colspan="3">'What's one thing the United Kingdom could learn from another country's drug policy?'
Pupils write their idea on a Post-it note or mini whiteboard.</td></tr>
<tr><td>Extension Activity</td><td>Creative challenge
On a world map (projected or printed), label key countries and their approach to drug laws (e.g. decriminalised, strict, tolerant).</td><td>Differentiation and Tips</td><td>Keyword cards or slides to support EAL/SEND pupils. Include terms like decriminalisation, zero tolerance, policy, harm reduction and stigma.
Provide a visual matching sheet if needed, with icons or flag cues for countries.</td></tr>
</table>

KS5 Tutor Time 4

<table>
<tr><td>Session Title</td><td>Mental Health and Substance Use: What Comes First?</td><td>Key Stage</td><td>3</td></tr>
<tr><td>Session Length</td><td>15–20 minutes</td><td>Linked Lesson Plan</td><td>KS3 Lesson 4
The Risks of Vaping and E-Cigarettes</td></tr>
<tr><td colspan="4">Intended Learning Focus</td></tr>
<tr><td colspan="4">To examine how substance use and mental health are linked and to reflect on ways to protect emotional well-being through healthy choices.</td></tr>
<tr><td>Resources Needed</td><td colspan="3">• Printed statements (optional)
• Post-its or whiteboards
• Paper and art supplies for the extension challenge (optional)</td></tr>
</table>

Warm-Up Question	**Use the following question as a discussion prompt:** 'Can poor mental health lead to substance use, or is it the other way around?' • Pupils reflect silently, then share in pairs. • Take a few responses as a class. **Discussion focus** • There's often a cycle or two-way relationship. • People may use substances to cope, which may worsen mental health over time.
Recap Activity	Give pairs or small groups a set of statements to sort into Cause, Effect, or Both. Examples include • Drinking to cope with stress. • Increased anxiety after regular cannabis use. • Substance withdrawal leading to depression. • Loneliness leading to increased alcohol use. • Poor sleep following stimulant misuse. **You could then ask** • Which examples were hard to place? • Can something be both a cause *and* an effect? • What can this tell us about the complexity of substance use and mental health?
Character and Values Reflection	**Discussion prompt** 'Why is self-awareness crucial in recognising when you need support?' You can use a quiet writing reflection using these sentence starters: • Being self-aware means . . . • I know I need support when . . . • I can check in with myself by . . . Option for pupils to share in pairs or whole group if appropriate.
Exit Question	**'What's one way to protect your mental health when facing stress?'** Get pupils to write one idea on a Post-it or in journals. Invite volunteers to share with the group or add to a classroom display titled 'Healthy Coping Habits.'

Extension Activity	**Creative Challenge** Create a class toolkit called 'Healthy Alternatives to Escape or Cope.' In small groups or individually, pupils suggest 1–2 healthy ways to manage stress, emotions, or low mood. Combine into a class 'Mental Health Toolkit' poster or digital slide.	**Differentiation and Tips**	Use sentence starters for all reflection prompts. Encourage peer talk for less confident speakers.

KS5 Tutor Time 5

Session Title	Testing the Limits: Drug Checks at Festivals	**Key Stage**	3
Session Length	15–20 minutes	**Linked Lesson Plan**	KS3 Lesson 5 Understanding Peer Pressure
Intended Learning Focus			
To engage in a balanced, respectful debate about drug testing at festivals, exploring the ethical, legal, and safety issues involved.			
Resources Needed	• Printed scenario cards or list for reading aloud • Post-it notes and pens • Display board or wall space for extension task (optional)		
Warm-Up Question	**'Should safety ever come before legality?'** Encourage individual silent reflection, then think-pair-share. Prompt ideas for examples: road safety, needle exchanges, supervised drug use spaces. Also, highlight the complexity of public health versus legal frameworks.		

<table>
<tr><td>Recap Activity</td><td colspan="3">Pupils work in pairs or small groups.
Half argue For drug testing at festivals, half argue Against.
Provide these prompts to structure thinking:
• Does drug testing at festivals save lives or send the wrong message?
• Is it a form of harm reduction or enabling illegal behaviour?
• Could testing reduce overdoses and contaminated drug risks?
• Who is responsible for keeping festival-goers safe – the individual, the organisers or public health services?
Invite one group from each side to share key points. If necessary, emphasise respectful listening and acknowledging complexity.</td></tr>
<tr><td>Character and Values Reflection</td><td colspan="3">Discussion prompt
'What role does fairness play in balancing public safety with personal choice?'
Get pupils to write a silent written response using sentence starters, if necessary:
• Fairness means . . .
• It's fair to test drugs at festivals when . . .
• Personal choice has limits when . . .</td></tr>
<tr><td>Exit Question</td><td colspan="3">'What's your position on drug testing at festivals, and why?'
Pupils write their personal stance with a one-sentence explanation. Responses can be kept private, shared in pairs or collected anonymously to gauge overall class views.</td></tr>
<tr><td>Extension Activity</td><td>Creative challenge
Create a campaign slogan for or against drug testing at festivals.
Pupils choose a stance (for or against) and create a clear, persuasive slogan in under 10 words.</td><td>Differentiation and Tips</td><td>Provide sentence starters for reflection and debate responses:
• I believe drug testing is/is not fair because . . .
• A benefit/risk of drug testing is . . .
• Allow written responses as an alternative to verbal debate.</td></tr>
</table>

KS5 Tutor Time 6

<table>
<tr><td rowspan="2">Session Title</td><td rowspan="2">Stay Smart, Stay Safe: Owning Your Choices in Social Spaces</td><td>Key Stage</td><td>5</td></tr>
<tr><td rowspan="2">Linked Lesson Plan</td><td rowspan="2">KS3 Lesson 6
Debate: Is Social Media as Harmful as Drugs and Alcohol for Mental Health?</td></tr>
<tr><td>Session Length</td><td>15–20 minutes</td></tr>
<tr><td colspan="4">Intended Learning Focus</td></tr>
<tr><td colspan="4">To reflect on practical strategies for staying safe, confident and in control in real-life social environments (parties, nightclubs, festivals), especially when substances may be involved.</td></tr>
<tr><td>Resources Needed</td><td colspan="3">• Statement cards or quiz slides
• Post-it notes or whiteboards
• Display materials for pledge poster</td></tr>
<tr><td>Warm-Up Question</td><td colspan="3">Use the following question as a discussion prompt:
'What helps someone stay true to their limits in a high-pressure setting?'
Think-pair-share
Pupils consider moments when peer influence can be strong.
Suggestions to prompt ideas include
• Having a trusted friend.
• Planning how much you'll drink (if at all).
• Knowing how to say no confidently.
• Setting a curfew or travel plan.</td></tr>
<tr><td>Recap Activity</td><td colspan="3">Read the following real-world scenarios aloud or display on the board:
1. Your friend mixes alcohol and pills at a party and starts acting confused.
2. Someone you don't know well offers you something – you're not sure what it is.
3. You lose your group at a busy festival, and your phone is nearly out of battery.
Pupils can discuss each scenario in small groups or pairs: 'What would you do in this situation?'
Encourage each group to share one strategy or key point with the class.
To support their discussion, you could ask
• How would you stay calm?
• What's a smart safety step you could take?
• Who would you ask for help or support?
Reinforce personal boundaries, looking after others and thinking ahead.</td></tr>
</table>

<table>
<tr><td>Character and Values Reflection</td><td colspan="3">Discussion prompt
'How does courage show up in social settings?'

Get pupils to do a silent written reflection or small-group discussion.

Use sentence starters, if necessary:
• Courage looks like . . .
• It takes courage to . . .
• Sometimes saying no is . . .

The key message here is that it often takes more courage to walk away or protect yourself than to fit in.</td></tr>
<tr><td>Exit Question</td><td colspan="3">'What's one personal boundary or safety plan you'll stick to in social spaces?'
Pupils write one personal rule or boundary they believe in (e.g. 'I will always stay with a friend I trust' or 'I will plan my way home before going out').

Offer the option to share voluntarily or keep responses private.</td></tr>
<tr><td>Extension Activity</td><td>Creative challenge
Class poster activity: 'Stay Smart at Festivals: 5 Golden Rules.'

As a class, brainstorm five key safety rules for attending festivals or parties (e.g. 'Don't leave your drink unattended'/'Set a check-in time with friends').</td><td>Differentiation and Tips</td><td>For pupils with social anxiety or prior experience of pressure, offer reassurance that boundaries are personal and valid.</td></tr>
</table>

9 Resources

DOI: 10.4324/9781003608998-9

Name: KS3 Lesson 1 Resource 1

Sorting Harmful Substances Pt. 1

Work in your pairs or groups to sort the substances below into the categories provided. Discuss each substance as you go. Think about whether it's legal or illegal, how it is used and how harmful it can be if misused.

______________	VS.	______________

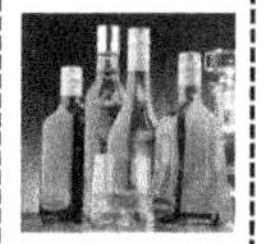
Alcohol

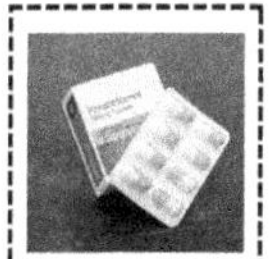
Paracetemol

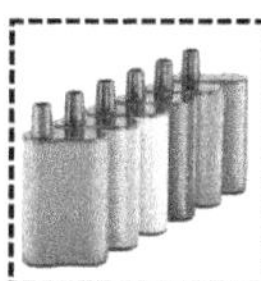
Vapes

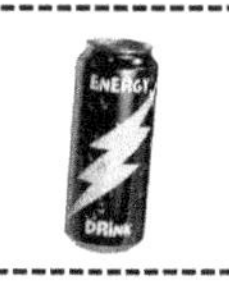

Energy Drinks

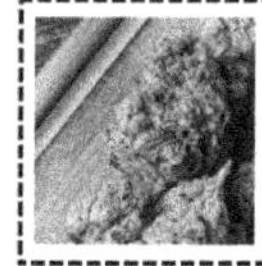
Cannabis

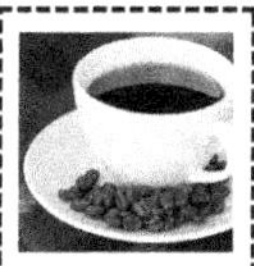
Caffeine

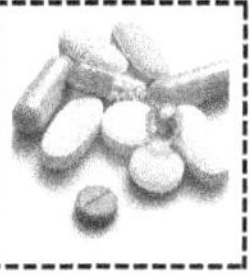
Antibiotics

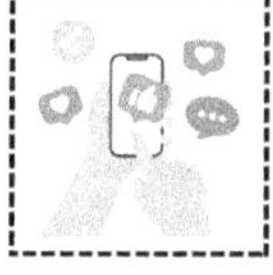
Social Media

Were there any substances your group disagreed about? Why?
Did any substances fit into more than one category?
Why is it important to understand how different substances are used and regulated?

Name:

KS3 Lesson 2 Resource 1

Sorting Harmful Substances Pt. 2

Work in pairs or small groups. Read through each item in the list and decide which category it fits best:

Medicinal
Recreational
Both

Medicinal	**VS.**	Recreational

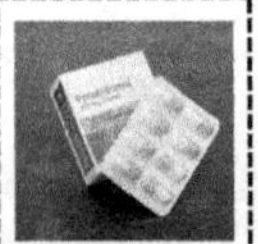

Paracetemol

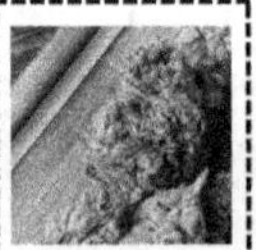

Cannabis

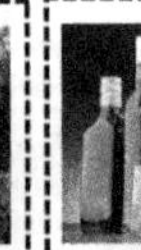

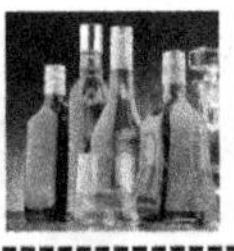

Alcohol

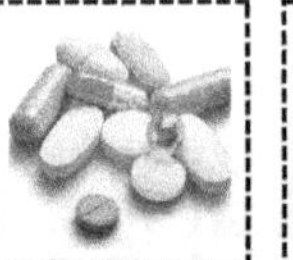

Antibiotics

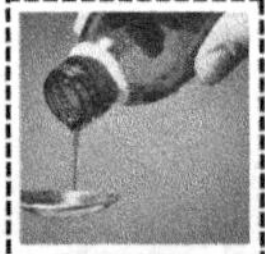

Cough Syrup

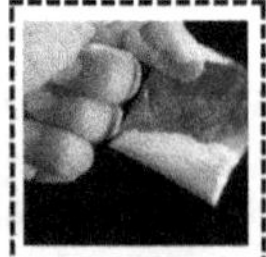

Cocaine

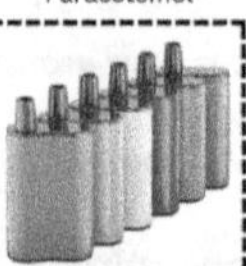

Vapes

Diazepam
(prescription sedative)

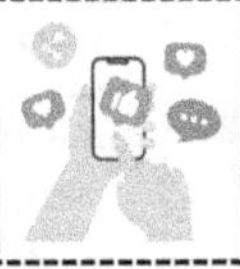

Social Media

Did anyone in your group disagree on where a substance belongs? Why?
Can a substance change category depending on how it's used?
Why is it important to understand how substances are classified?

Role Play Scenarios

Scenario 1

You're at a friend's house party and someone you've just met offers you a vape. They say, "It's just for fun, everyone's doing it," and pass it to you in front of a group of people. Some of your friends are already vaping, and they're watching to see what you'll do.

Scenario 2

Before a big football match, a couple of your teammates hand out energy drinks and tell everyone it'll give them a boost. One friend says, "You'll never keep up without one." You've never tried them before and feel unsure, but you don't want to let the team down.

Scenario 3

At a birthday get-together, most people are having a drink. When you turn down an alcoholic drink and ask for something else, someone jokes, "Come on, don't be boring!" Others laugh along, and you feel awkward and left out – even though you're not sure you want to drink.

Scenario 4

Your teacher pressures you to fight someone to prove you're brave.

During a heated moment in class, a teacher jokingly (but seriously) says, "If you're so tough, why don't you fight him after school and show us what you've got?" You're shocked. This isn't something you expected an adult to say. Other students laugh awkwardly, and you feel stuck between wanting to prove yourself and knowing this isn't right.

Name: ______________________ KS3 Lesson 6 Resource 1

Analysis Framework

Coping Under Pressure: Choices and Consequences

1 What is dopamine and how does it relate to addiction?

____

____

____

2 What are the known mental health effects of social media

____

____

3 How do drugs and alcohol affect mental health?

____

____

____

4 Can social media be used in healthy ways? Give examples.

____

____

____

____

KS4 Lesson 5 Resource 1

DEBATE PLANNING SHEET

GROUP PARTICIPANTS

____

____

____

FOR/ AGAINST

TOPIC QUESTION:

Is Social Media as Harmful as Drugs and Alcohol for Mental Health?

ARGUMENT	SUPPORTING EVIDENCE

CLOSING STATEMENT

Name: KS4 Lesson 1 Resource 1

Substance Effects Quiz

What Do You Know About Common Substances?

Instructions:

Answer the questions as best as you can. This is not a test! It is just a way to start thinking and talking about the topic. You can work alone or discuss in pairs/groups.

Which of the following substances is legal for adults to buy and use in the UK?
a) Alcohol
b) Tobacco
c) Cannabis
d) All of the above
e) Only a and b

What is the legal age for buying alcohol in the UK?
a) 16
b) 18
c) 21
d) There is no legal age

What does nicotine (in tobacco and vapes) do to the body?
a) It calms the brain and helps sleep
b) It makes the heart beat faster and can be addictive
c) It helps fight infections
d) It builds muscle

What short-term effects can alcohol have on the brain and body?
(Tick all that apply)
□ Slower reaction time
□ Improved memory
□ Poor decision-making
□ Blurred vision

True or False:
Smoking cannabis is completely safe because it's natural.
□ True
□ False

Which of the following can be risks of using cannabis regularly?
a) Improved concentration
b) Memory problems
c) Motivation loss
d) Better fitness

Name: KS3 Lesson 1 Resource 2

Substance Cards

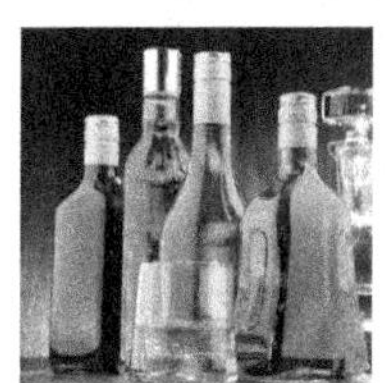 Alcohol	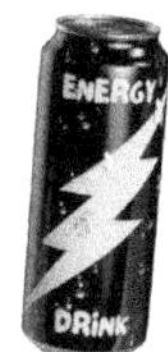 Energy Drinks	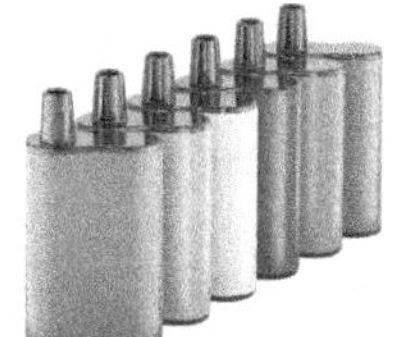 Vapes
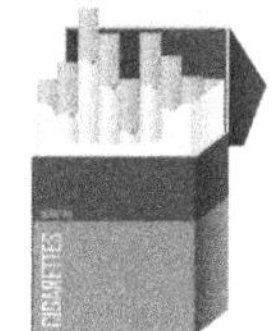 Cigarettes	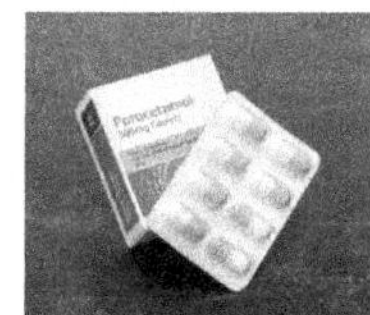 Paracetemol	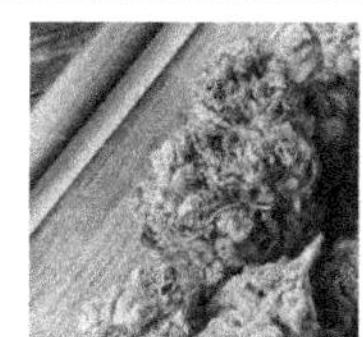 Cannabis

Name: KS3 Lesson 1 Resource 2

Effect Cards

Addiction	Anxiety
Liver Damage	Lung Damage
Poor Concentration	Sleep Disruption
Risky Behaviour	Impaired Judgement
Aggression	Financial Problems
Legal Trouble	Overdose Risk
Depression	Increased Heart Rate
Peer Pressure	Hallucinations

Name: ______________________ KS4 Lesson 2 Resource 1

Real or Not? Sorting Everyday Pressures

Instructions:

In pairs or small groups, read each scenario carefully.

Your task is to sort each one into one of the following categories:

- Realistic pressure/influence – This could genuinely happen in real life.
- Exaggerated or unlikely – It's not something that would usually happen or is very unrealistic.
- Unsure – You're not sure if this could happen or not.

Scenario 1

Your friend dares you to vape at lunch, saying everyone's doing it.

You're sitting outside during lunch when your friend pulls out a vape and passes it to you. They laugh and say, "Come on, just try it — everyone's doing it now." A few others in the group are watching, waiting to see what you'll do. You feel nervous and unsure — you don't want to look uncool, but you're not sure you really want to try it.

Scenario 2

An influencer posts a photo of a 'perfect' body and says, 'No excuses!'

You're scrolling through social media when you see a fitness influencer showing off their toned body with the caption, "No excuses — if I can do it, so can you." They have thousands of likes and comments praising their appearance. You start to feel self-conscious and wonder if you're doing enough to look that way, even though their lifestyle seems unrealistic.

Scenario 3

A classmate suggests bunking class to hang out, saying it's no big deal.

It's the last lesson of the day, and a classmate leans over and whispers, "Let's sneak out and chill at the park. It's just one class, and we're not doing anything important anyway." They make it sound like harmless fun, and you know others have done it without getting caught. Still, something doesn't sit right with you.

Scenario 4

Your teacher pressures you to fight someone to prove you're brave.

During a heated moment in class, a teacher jokingly (but seriously) says, "If you're so tough, why don't you fight him after school and show us what you've got?" You're shocked. This isn't something you expected an adult to say. Other students laugh awkwardly, and you feel stuck between wanting to prove yourself and knowing this isn't right.

Name: ____________________ KS4 Lesson 2 Resource 2

Real or Not? Sorting Everyday Pressures

Instructions:

In pairs or small groups, read each scenario carefully and then complete your question sheet.

Scenario 1

A friend dares you to vape at a party.

You're at a party when a friend hands you a vape and says, "Come on, just try it...I dare you!" Others are watching and waiting to see what you'll do.

Scenario 2

You feel bad after seeing filtered selfies online.

You're scrolling through social media and see filtered selfies of people looking perfect. You start comparing yourself and feel like you don't measure up.

Scenario 3

An influencer promotes a 'magic' weight-loss tea.

An influencer you follow posts about a "miracle" tea that promises quick weight loss without exercise or diet changes. They claim it changed their life and urge their followers to buy it.

Scenario 4

Your mates make fun of someone who doesn't drink.

At a social event, a few people laugh at someone who chooses not to drink alcohol, calling them "boring" and "no fun."

Scenario 5

You see a TikTok challenge encouraging risky behaviour.

A trending TikTok video shows people doing a risky challenge, like taking too many energy drinks or doing a dangerous stunt. It has thousands of likes and comments.

Scenario 6

Someone tells you you're boring if you don't take something 'just once'.

During a hangout, someone offers you a pill or drink and says, "It's no big deal – just try it once. You're boring if you don't."

Name: ____________________ KS4 Lesson 2 Resource 2

Real or Not? Sorting Everyday Pressures

Question and Answer Sheet

Scenario ______
·What's happening in this scenario?

·How could this situation make someone feel?

·What's a confident or positive way to respond?

Scenario ______
·What's happening in this scenario?

·How could this situation make someone feel?

·What's a confident or positive way to respond?

Scenario ______
·What's happening in this scenario?

·How could this situation make someone feel?

·What's a confident or positive way to respond?

Name: ______________________ KS4 Lesson 3 Resource 1

Coping Under Pressure: Choices and Consequences

Instructions:

In pairs or small groups, read each scenario carefully.

Scenario 1

Aiden is in Year 11 and feeling the pressure of upcoming exams. He's been working late most nights, barely sleeping, and says his mind is constantly racing. At weekends, he goes to parties and drinks alcohol, telling his friends it helps him "switch off" and forget about school for a while. He doesn't see it as a big deal – just something to help him cope.

Scenario 2

Sophie often feels alone at school and finds it hard to connect with others. She spends more time online where she chats with a friend she met in a private group. One day, the friend says they sometimes take pills that "make you feel better when you're down" and offers to send Sophie some. Sophie is tempted – she wants to feel happy, but she's not sure if it's safe or what the pills even are.

Scenario 3

Liam's home life is tense. His parents argue almost every night, and he often feels caught in the middle. At school, he tries to act like everything's fine, but inside he feels anxious and on edge. One day, a friend offers him a vape, saying it helps them relax. Liam tries it and starts vaping regularly, thinking it helps him stay calm when things get stressful at home.

Scenario 4

Priya is a caring older sister who takes on a lot of responsibility at home, helping with meals, school runs, and looking after her younger sibling. At the same time, school is getting more demanding, and she feels like she's always behind. She doesn't feel like she has time for herself, so she starts skipping meals and sleeping during the day to avoid everything. She hasn't told anyone how she's feeling.

Name: ____________________

KS4 Lesson 3 Resource 2

Analysis Framework

Coping Under Pressure: Choices and Consequences

1 What emotion/s is the person experiencing?

____

____

2 What substance or behaviour are they turning to?

____

____

3 Why do you think they chose that coping strategy?

____

____

4 What are the short- and long-term consequences?

____

____

5 What healthier coping strategies could they use instead?

____

____

6 How could a friend or trusted adult help?

____

____

Name: ____________________ KS4 Lesson 4 Resource 1

When Choices Impact Relationships: Real-Life Case Studies

Instructions:

In pairs or small groups, read each scenario carefully.

Scenario 1

Ethan is 15 and recently started drinking alcohol at the weekends. It began with small amounts at parties, but now he sometimes drinks alone when he's stressed or bored. His mum has noticed a change in him – he's more distant, moody, and his grades have started to slip. One evening, she finds empty bottles in his room and confronts him. Ethan gets angry and defensive, shouting that she's overreacting. Their relationship becomes tense, and Ethan starts avoiding her altogether.

Scenario 2

Layla, 16, has been smoking cannabis with a new group of older friends after school. At first, it made her feel relaxed and accepted. But lately, she's been cancelling plans with her best friend, Mia, to hang out with the new group instead. Mia feels hurt and left out. When she brings it up, Layla shrugs it off and tells her to "stop being so dramatic." Their friendship starts to fade, and Layla becomes more withdrawn and forgetful in class.

Scenario 3

Josh is 15 and has recently taken up vaping, saying it helps him stay calm during exams. His girlfriend, Zara, doesn't like it. She's worried about his health and how dependent he's become on it. She's brought it up a few times, but Josh brushes it off, saying, "It's not that deep – it's better than smoking." They begin arguing more often, and Zara starts pulling away. Josh feels frustrated but doesn't think his vaping is really the problem.

Scenario 4

Amira, 14, has been drinking several energy drinks a day to stay awake after long nights gaming. Her sleep pattern is all over the place, and she often turns up to school tired and irritable. Her favourite teacher, Mr. Collins, notices she's no longer contributing in class and seems distracted. He gently asks if she's okay, but Amira shrugs and says she's "just tired." He offers support, but she pushes him away, embarrassed and unsure how to talk about what's really going on.

Response Sheet

KS4 Lesson 4 Resource 2

Scenario 1	What is happening in this situation? How is the relationship being affected? What advice or healthy support could help this person or their relationship?
Scenario 2	What is happening in this situation? How is the relationship being affected? What advice or healthy support could help this person or their relationship?
Scenario 3	What is happening in this situation? How is the relationship being affected? What advice or healthy support could help this person or their relationship?
Scenario 4	What is happening in this situation? How is the relationship being affected? What advice or healthy support could help this person or their relationship?

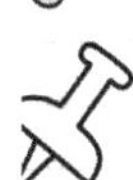
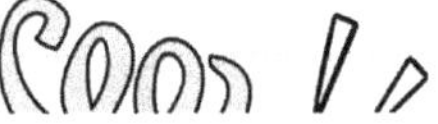

KS4 Lesson 5 Resource 1

DEBATE PLANNING SHEET

GROUP PARTICIPANTS

FOR/ AGAINST

TOPIC QUESTION:

ARGUMENT	SUPPORTING EVIDENCE

CLOSING STATEMENT

Name: ____________________

KS4 Lesson 5 Resource 2

Reflection Sheet

1 What was your original opinion about banning smoking?

____

____

2 Did today's debate change your opinion? Why or why not?

____

____

3 What was one argument you heard that made you think differently?

____

____

4 What's your final view on whether smoking should be banned? Explain your reasoning.

____

____

____

____

____

____

____

____

SCENARIO 1

Tyler, 16, was at a party when police arrived in response to noise complaints. During a search, officers found a small bag of cannabis in his pocket. He admitted it was his and said he brought it to "help him relax." Tyler received a youth caution, which now shows up on certain types of background checks. His school found out and suspended him for two weeks. His parents were furious, and a family holiday was cancelled. Tyler later found out he may have to declare the caution on future job or college applications.

SCENARIO 2

Ella, 17, was struggling with revision and borrowed ADHD medication from her older cousin, thinking it would help her concentrate. She didn't tell anyone, but a teacher noticed unusual behaviour and reported it to the safeguarding team. When the truth came out, Ella was given a formal warning by the school and missed her mock exams while investigations were ongoing. Her parents were disappointed, and her friends began treating her differently. Though she wasn't arrested, the experience damaged her confidence and reputation at school.

SCENARIO 3

Sam, 15, was caught by police giving a classmate a vape pen filled with cannabis oil in a shopping centre car park. CCTV and texts confirmed he'd done it before. He was arrested and charged with intent to supply a controlled substance. Sam now has a youth criminal record. He had planned to apply for a college engineering course, but the college has placed his application on hold pending the outcome of the case. His friendship group has split, with some distancing themselves from the situation.

SCENARIO 4

Mia, 16, was found by security staff at a local music festival with several nitrous oxide canisters in her bag. She had planned to share them with friends "just for fun." Security handed her over to police, and she was issued a community resolution. Photos taken at the event were later posted online, and a teacher recognised her. The school gave Mia a warning and removed her from a leadership role she had worked hard for. Her parents were upset, and her relationship with a close friend deteriorated after a falling-out over the incident.

Response Sheet

KS4 Lesson 6 Resource 2

Scenario 1	What happened in this scenario? What were the short- and long-term legal/social consequences? How did this affect the person's life, relationships, or opportunities? What alternative choices could have been made, and what might the outcomes have been?
Scenario 2	What happened in this scenario? What were the short- and long-term legal/social consequences? How did this affect the person's life, relationships, or opportunities? What alternative choices could have been made, and what might the outcomes have been?
Scenario 3	What happened in this scenario? What were the short- and long-term legal/social consequences? How did this affect the person's life, relationships, or opportunities? What alternative choices could have been made, and what might the outcomes have been?
Scenario 4	What happened in this scenario? What were the short- and long-term legal/social consequences? How did this affect the person's life, relationships, or opportunities? What alternative choices could have been made, and what might the outcomes have been?

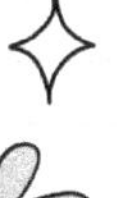

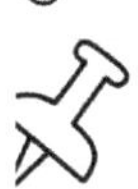

Name: KS5 Lesson 1 Resource 1

Case File Worksheet

Examine your assigned substance through these key lenses

Substance:

Physical health effects (short- and long-term)

Mental health impacts (e.g. anxiety, depression, psychosis)

Legal status and implications (possession, supply, sentencing)

Cultural/media representation, or recent debates (optional)

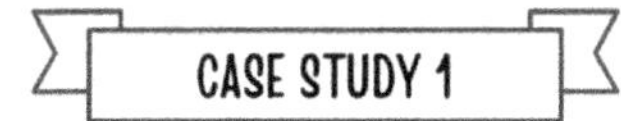

CASE STUDY 1

Jack, 17, started smoking cigarettes at 14, after trying one with an older cousin. Despite several attempts to quit, he finds himself irritable, anxious, and unable to focus without smoking. His dad and grandfather were both long-term smokers, and Jack's parents believe "addiction runs in the family." Jack knows it's bad for his health but says the cravings feel stronger than his willpower. Even nicotine patches didn't help for long – he relapsed after just a few days.

SCENARIO 2

Amber, 18, began using cannabis regularly after her parents separated. She says it helps her "shut off" the anxiety and sadness she feels most days. Over time, it became part of her daily routine. She often smokes alone in her room and says it's the only thing that helps her sleep. Her school attendance is dropping, and her motivation has declined. When asked if she's addicted, Amber says, "I could stop if I wanted to – I just don't want to feel worse."

SCENARIO 3

Leo, 19, is at university and drinks heavily on weekends with his friends. What began as occasional drinking escalated into regular binge episodes. He says alcohol helps him be more confident and social. His dad also has a history of alcohol problems, and Leo grew up in a home where heavy drinking was normalised. Since moving away for uni, he's felt lonely and stressed, and uses alcohol to "have fun" and escape. His grades are slipping, and his friends are starting to worry about his behaviour.

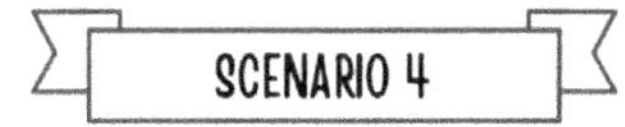

SCENARIO 4

Priya, 17, was prescribed strong painkillers after a sports injury. Even after her physical pain eased, she continued using the medication to manage stress and help her sleep. She's become increasingly reliant and now finds it difficult to go a day without them. Her mum is worried and has started monitoring her prescriptions. Priya insists she's "still in pain," but also admits that the pills help her "feel calm." She's now withdrawn from her sports team and misses social events.

Name: ____________________ KS5 Lesson 3 Resource 1

Analysis Framework

Country:

1 What is the country's approach to drug use and policy?

____

____

2 What impact has this had on the population or public health?

____

____

____

____

3 What social, cultural, legal or economic factors might explain the drug use rates?

____

4 What are the strengths and weaknesses of this country's approach?

____

____

5 Extension: How does this compare with what you know about drug policy in the UK or elsewhere?

____

____

____

SCENARIO 1

Alex is 19 and in his first year of university. Although he was excited to start a new chapter, he's found the transition overwhelming. He struggles with social anxiety and feels constantly on edge in group settings or seminars. To help himself "feel normal," Alex drinks before nights out and sometimes before classes. What started as a coping mechanism has led to frequent hangovers, missed deadlines, and a growing sense of isolation. Lately, Alex has noticed his mood dropping and says he feels numb most of the time.

SCENARIO 2

Zara is 21 and has recently been diagnosed with bipolar disorder. During her manic episodes, she feels invincible and often takes risks, including using recreational drugs at parties. During depressive phases, she isolates herself and sometimes uses substances to numb the pain. Zara has been prescribed mood stabilisers, but she sometimes skips doses when she feels "fine." Her partner has noticed the changes in her behaviour and is beginning to feel unsafe and confused about how to help.

SCENARIO 3

Marcus, 18, experienced emotional neglect and trauma in childhood, which he rarely talks about. After a minor car accident, he was prescribed strong painkillers. He quickly noticed how they also dulled his emotional pain, and he continued to take them even after his injury healed. Now, he feels dependent on the pills to get through the day. He's withdrawn from friends, dropped out of college, and says he doesn't "feel anything unless he's on something."

SCENARIO 4

Lily is 17 and has been in and out of support services for alcohol misuse over the past two years. She initially began drinking at parties to fit in, but it quickly became a way to block out negative thoughts and feelings. Despite periods of sobriety, she often relapses when life becomes overwhelming. Each time she relapses, she feels more ashamed and hopeless. Her confidence is low, and she believes she'll "never be good enough" to recover or have a better future.

KS5 Lesson 5 Resource 1

DEBATE PLANNING SHEET

GROUP PARTICIPANTS

FOR/ AGAINST

TOPIC QUESTION:

ARGUMENT	SUPPORTING EVIDENCE

CLOSING STATEMENT

SCENARIO 1

You're at a music festival with your friends when one of them admits they've taken a pill from someone they didn't know. Not long after, they start feeling really unwell, dizzy, nauseous and panicked. They beg you not to tell anyone, saying they'll be fine soon and don't want to get into trouble. You're not sure whether to believe them or how serious it is.

SCENARIO 2

You're in a club and someone you've just met offers to get you a drink. They return with it already poured, saying, "Here you go!" You didn't see the drink being made and feel a bit unsure – but they seem friendly, and you don't want to seem rude or overreact.

SCENARIO 3

It's late and your group is invited to an after-party by some people you barely know. You're tired, uncomfortable and not sure you want to stay but your friends are really keen and tell you to just "chill and go with the flow." You feel pressured to stay, even though something about it doesn't feel right.

SCENARIO 4

You're hanging out with friends when one of them offers you something to take – a pill or something to smoke – saying, "Come on, just try it once, everyone's doing it." They laugh it off when you hesitate and say you're being boring. You don't want to feel left out, but you're also not sure about it.

Name:

Party Safety Plan

Pre-Event Prep:

- ______________________________
- ______________________________
- ______________________________

During the Event:

____

____

____

____

If Things Go Wrong

____

____

____

____

____

____

____

____

Post-Event:

____

____

____

____

____

____

____

References

Action on Smoking and Health (ASH). (2021). *Facts at a Glance*. [online]. https://ash.org.uk/resources/view/facts-at-a-glance.

Adfam. (n.d.). *Family support services*. https://adfam.org.uk/for-families/.

Centre for Public Health, Faculty of Health, & Applied Social Science, Liverpool John Moores University. (2011, August). *A summary of the health harms of drugs*. Department of Health and National Treatment Agency for Substance Misuse. https://assets.publishing.service.gov.uk/media/5a74ebfc40f0b65c0e845947/dh_129674.pdfE. Last accessed: 5 April 2025.

Department for Education (DfE). (2019). *Relationships education, relationships and sex education (RSE) and health education*. GOV.UK. https://www.gov.uk/government/publications/relationships-education-relationships-and-sex-education-rse-and-health-education. Last accessed: 31 May 2025.

Department for Education (DfE). (2021, September 13). *Statutory guidance: Physical health and mental wellbeing (primary and secondary)*. Department for Education. https://www.gov.uk/government/publications/relationships-education-relationships-and-sex-education-rse-and-health-education/physical-health-and-mental-wellbeing-primary-and-secondary. Last accessed: 22 February 2025.

Department for Education (DfE). (2024). *Keeping children safe in education: Statutory guidance for schools and colleges*. https://assets.publishing.service.gov.uk/media/66d7301b9084b18b95709f75/Keeping_children_safe_in_education_2024.pdf.

Department for Education, & Association of Chief Police Officers. (2012). *DfE and ACPO drug advice for schools* [report]. https://

assets.publishing.service.gov.uk/media/5a75b67a40f0b67b3d5c8a26/drug_advice_for_schools.pdf.

Education Endowment Foundation (EEF). (2021). *Guest blog: Retrieval practice – a common good or just commonplace?* [online]. EEF. https://educationendowmentfoundation.org.uk/news/guest-blog-retrieval-practice-a-common-good-or-just-commonplace-2. Last accessed: 2 June 2025.

European Commission. (n.d.a). *Harmful substances: Definitions and classifications*. European Commission.

European Commission. (n.d.b). https://ec.europa.eu/taxation_customs/dds2/SAMANCTA/EN/Safety/HazardousSubstances_EN.htm#:~:text=A%20hazardous%20substance%20is%20any,substances%20which%20are%20being%20transported. Last accessed: 22 February 2025.

FRANK. (n.d.). *Talk to FRANK*. https://www.talktofrank.com/. Last accessed: 11 May 2025.

HM Government. (2017). *2017 drug strategy*. [online]. https://assets.publishing.service.gov.uk/media/5a82b5a2e5274a2e87dc2966/Drug_strategy_2017.PDF. Last accessed: 1 July 2025.

HM Government. (n.d.a). *Alcohol and young people: The law*. GOV.UK. https://www.gov.uk/alcohol-young-people-law.

HM Government. (n.d.b). *Penalties for drug possession, supply and production*. GOV.UK. https://www.gov.uk/penalties-drug-possession-dealing. Last accessed: 23 April 2025.

Manchester Metropolitan University. (2022). *New drug trends: Research findings and implications for young people*. https://www.mmu.ac.uk/research/our-impact/case-studies/new-drug-trends. Last accessed: 22 February 2025.

Martin, K. (2023). *3 strategies to get all pupils participating*. [online]. Edutopia. https://www.edutopia.org/article/strategies-increasing-student-participation/. Last accessed: 2 June 2025.

Mental Health Foundation. (2021). *Drugs and mental health*. Mental Health Foundation. https://www.mentalhealth.org.uk/explore-mental-health/a-z-topics/drugs-and-mental-health. Last accessed: 23 February 2025.

Mentor UK. (n.d.). *Information and advice for schools and communities*. https://www.mentoruk.org.uk/information-and-advice/information-for-schools-and-communities/. Last accessed: 2 May 2025.

National Health Service (NHS). (2020a). *Better health*. [online]. nhs.uk. https://www.nhs.uk/better-health/. Last accessed: 18 June 2025.

National Health Service (NHS). (2020b). *Quit smoking – better heath*. [online]. http://www.nhs.uk/smokefree. Last accessed: 18 June 2025.

National Health Service (NHS). (n.d.). *Young people and vaping*. NHS. https://www.nhs.uk/better-health/quit-smoking/help-others-quit/young-people-and-vaping/.

National Institute for Health and Care Excellence. (2019). *Evidence review of the acceptability of universal school-based alcohol interventions*. Draft for Consultation. Public Health – Internal Guideline Development Team.

National Institute on Drug Abuse. (2021). *Stigma and discrimination*. [online]. National Institute on Drug Abuse. https://nida.nih.gov/research-topics/stigma-discrimination.

NHS Digital. (2023). *Statistics on public health: Part 5 – other data sources*. https://digital.nhs.uk/data-and-information/publications/statistical/statistics-on-public-health/2023/part-5-other-data-sources. Last accessed: 2 May 2025.

NSPCC. (2023). *Parental substance misuse: Protecting children living in families affected by substance misuse*. NSPCC Learning. https://learning.nspcc.org.uk/children-and-families-at-risk/parental-substance-misuse.

Office for Health Improvement & Disparities. (2024, January). *UK report on substance misuse in young people*. UK Government. https://www.gov.uk/government/statistics/substance-misuse-treatment-for-young-people-2022-to-2023/young-peoples-substance-misuse-treatment-statistics-2022-to-2023-report. Last accessed: 22 February 2025.

PSHE Association. (2016). *Key principles of effective prevention education*. https://pshe-association.org.uk/evidence-and-research-key-principles-of-effective-prevention-education. Last accessed: 1 July 2025.

PSHE Association. (2021). *Drug and alcohol education: Effective approaches in PSHE education*. https://pshe-association.org.uk/drugeducation.

PSHE Association. (2025). *Drug education for pupils with SEND*. [online]. https://pshe-association.org.uk/resource/drugs-alcohol-lessons-send. Last accessed: 31 May 2025.

PSHE Association. (n.d.). *Drug and alcohol education*. https://pshe-association.org.uk/drugeducation. Last accessed: 2 May 2025.

Public Health England. (2018). *Improving young people's health and wellbeing: A framework for public health*. https://www.gov.uk/government/publications/improving-young-peoples-health-and-wellbeing-a-framework-for-public-health. Last accessed: 8 May 2025.

UK Addiction Treatment Centres. (2021). *Why is cannabis use so prevalent in young communities? | UKAT blog*. [online]. UK Addiction Treatment Centres. https://www.ukat.co.uk/blog/adolescents/cannabis-young-communities/. Last accessed: 1 July 2025.

UK Addiction Treatment Centres. (n.d.). *Substance abuse for children | recognising addiction in children*. [online]. https://www.ukat.co.uk/help-guides/recognise-substance-abuse-for-children/. Last accessed: 27 May 2025.

We Are with You. (n.d.). *Supporting people with drug, alcohol or mental health issues*. https://www.wearewithyou.org.uk/. Last accessed: 11 May 2025.

YoungMinds. (2024). *Drugs and alcohol: Guide for parents*. https://www.youngminds.org.uk/parent/parents-a-z-mental-health-guide/drugs-and-alcohol/. Last accessed: 11 May 2025.

Journals

Arain, M., Haque, M., Johal, L., Mathur, P., Nel, W., Rais, A., Sandhu, R., & Sharma, S. (2013). Maturation of the adolescent brain. *Neuropsychiatric Disease and Treatment*, [online], 9(9), 449–461. https://doi.org/10.2147/ndt.s39776.

Squeglia, L.M., Jacobus, J., & Tapert, S.F. (2009). The influence of substance use on adolescent brain development. *Clinical EEG and Neuroscience*, [online], 40(1), 31–38. https://doi.org/10.1177/155005940904000110.

Waples, L., Carlisle, V.R., & Maynard, O.M. (2023). "They're doing it anyway, let's have a conversation about it": Exploring student and stakeholder attitudes towards drug education programmes for university students. *Drugs: Education, Prevention and Policy*, 1–10. https://doi.org/10.1080/09687637.2023.2181148.

Factsheet

Why you should talk with your child about alcohol and other drugs parents have a significant influence in their children's decisions to experiment with alcohol and other drugs. (n.d.). https://library.samhsa.gov/sites/default/files/sma18–5076_0.pdf. Last accessed: 31 May 2025.

Index

Note: Page numbers in *italics* indicate a figure on the corresponding page.

www.ingramcontent.com/pod-product-compliance
Lightning Source LLC
LaVergne TN
LVHW010648110826
845149LV00014B/2992

* 9 7 8 1 0 4 1 0 0 2 7 0 3 *